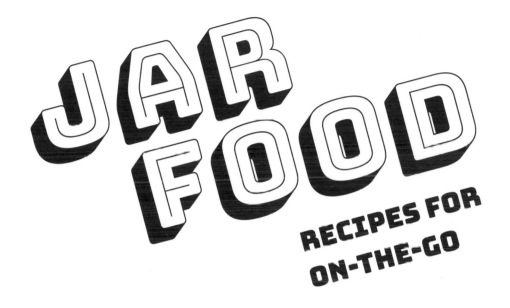

JAR FOOD

RECIPES FOR ON-THE-GO

**DOMINIQUE
ELOÏSE
ALEXANDER**

PAVILION

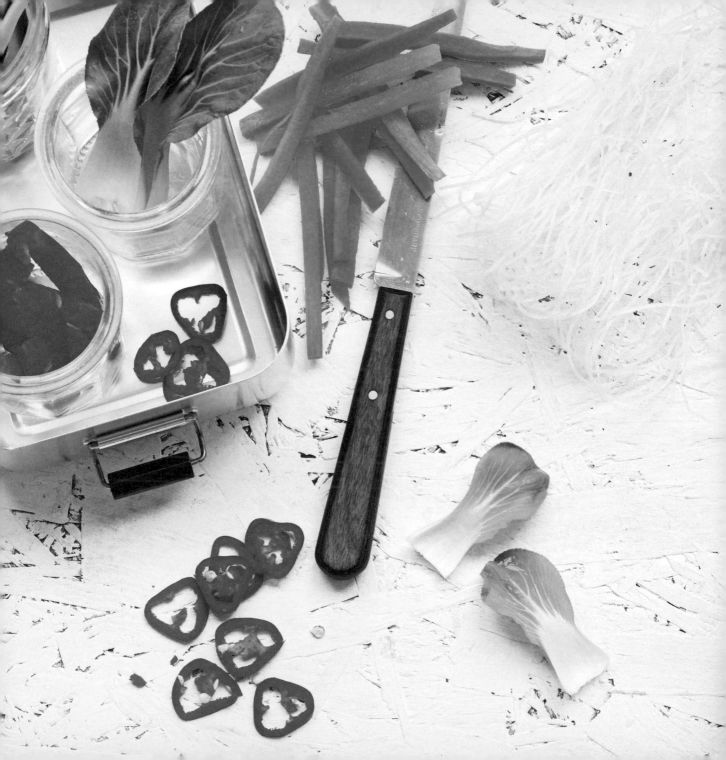

CONTENTS

INTRODUCTION

For me, having the autonomy to create one's own food has always been exciting. From cooking meals for my brother and myself after school to challenging myself through university to try different ingredients every week and embracing the joy that home cooking could bring. That love has only grown in the past few years and as I have got busier, my cooking has had to keep up. *Jar Foods* is a way of taking great wholesome food with you every day whatever you are doing. Whether it is having breakfast on the go or taking ten minutes for a breath of fresh air and a quick snack in the afternoon to refocus, these recipes will allow you to nourish yourself with minimal effort.

Eating in-season foods is very important to me and is a great way to keep costs down when shopping for your fruit and veg. The recipes in this book take you through all the seasons, so if you are struggling to find something at a particular time of year, take a moment to think what that adds to the jar and if there's something you can see that has those same flavour elements. I have included some suggestions throughout the book, but asking your greengrocer or having a quick search online before you shop can be just as easy to find alternatives and ideas.

Alternative diets are also something I am passionate about. Great food is only great if lots of people can enjoy it. The wonderful thing about making your own breakfasts and lunches is that you can completely personalise them based on your tastes. These recipes are crying out to be chopped and changed with any ingredient you prefer. The majority of the recipes in this book are either vegetarian or vegan (or with optional ingredients to make them so) and I have also made sure to include plenty of gluten- and dairy-free options as well. This variety is the true essence of *Jar Foods,* having deliciously easy food ready to take with you when you need it, fuelling you for all that your life gives you.

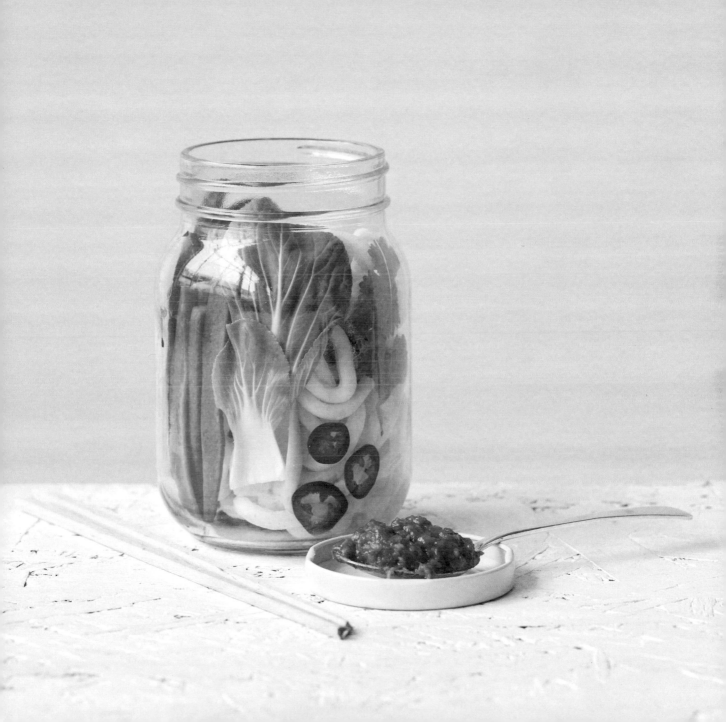

WHY JAR FOODS?

Jars are first and foremost all around us. Many of these recipes can be made with any leftover jars you have although for some recipes it may be worth investing in some slightly larger ones to fit in all the ingredients! Glass is more easily recyclable than plastic and doing anything to reduce the dreaded Tupperware lid search on a frantic morning can only be a good thing. Jars are also gorgeous to look at. It's easy to see in your refrigerator exactly what you have as well as allowing you to pick your favourite bits out with your fork easily when eating.

My mum always said to us 'a Sunday well spent brings a week of content' and I think that is never truer than when talking about batch cooking. It not only keeps costs down but also makes life so much easier. By spending a couple of hours on a Sunday making a few breakfasts and lunches for the week ahead you leave yourself your weekday mornings and evenings free to do whatever you like without having to worry. In each recipe I have made a note of how long they keep in the refrigerator to help with planning. Sometimes I like to make a slightly more complex recipe on a Sunday for Monday, Tuesday and Wednesday, then pick a quicker one to make on Wednesday evening for the rest of the week. Fridays can be a bit of a struggle if there is not much left in the refrigerator, so I hope the recipes in this book give you plenty of ideas for just how easy it is to put together a meal in a jar.

Each recipe makes 1 jar's worth and I have specified the size of the jar so you can compare it to what you have at home – the easiest way to do this is fill it with water then pour it into a measuring jug/cup. Some of the recipes do need a larger jar to fit in all of the lovely ingredients, so it might be worth investing in two or three jars so you can prep ahead for the week. All the recipes are simple enough to multiply easily as needed and the main meals are equally delicious as dinners both on the go and at home for a few hungry housemates.

ESSENTIAL KIT

The basic bits you will need to make your life easier are:

1 x 1 litre/34fl oz jar (for a large batch of granola)
3 x 500ml/18fl oz jars (perfect for breakfasts)
2 x 700ml/25 fl oz jars (best for main meals)
4 x 250ml/9fl oz jars (great for snacks)
4 x 100ml/3½fl oz jars (these little guys so cute for puddings)

I like both screw-top and rubber-sealed preserving jars – there really isn't a best one. Tiny rubber-sealed jars are great for dressings to avoid any spillage en route and double up as great pudding pots.

Wide neck funnel: no spillage whatsoever and keeps everything simple when filling up your jars.

Salad spinner: I was lost without one and now I use it all the time. It saves so much time when putting together jars.

REHEATING TIPS

If you are reheating your jars at work there are a couple of things to consider. To keep it super-easy if you have a microwave I would suggest using screw-top jars, as they are easy to remove the metal from and you can eat straight out of them. About 4–5 minutes on medium heat setting should be enough and it's always worth stirring halfway through cooking to help things along. If you are heating in the oven with either type of jar, remember to remove any rubber seals so they don't melt. I usually preheat the oven to 160°C/325°F/Gas mark 3 for about 20 minutes to ensure everything inside is piping hot. Whatever reheating method you use, **please** use proper oven gloves (mitts) or a triple-folded dry tea towel to remove the jars. Glass gets so hot and I'd hate for you to burn yourselves or drop your lovingly prepared meals. Leave them to stand at room temperature for a couple of minutes post-heating before either turning out into a bowl or plate or diving straight in with your fork.

MEAL PLANNER

Lots of these recipes you'll notice have easily interchangeable ingredients, such as the veg, making them able to be entirely your own. This also means that if you've got a glut of something to use up you can find a few different ways of making them taste great. For example, carrots are fantastic in the Burrito Jar, Asian Noodle Soup and the Sushi Jar. They even make up one of the main root vegetables for the Winter Warmer Soup – another great recipe to use up whatever veg you have left in the bottom of your fridge at the end of the week. In this sample weekly meal planner for days when you are eating away from home, the recipes use similar ingredients but yield different meals.

	MONDAY	TUESDAY
BREAKFAST	Basic Granola (see page 14)	Grilled Stone Fruit Jar with Vanilla and Almonds (see page 19)
LUNCH	Sushi Jar (see page 32)	Burrito Jar (see page 44)
SNACK	Nut Butter and Fruit Crisps (see page 63)	Chocolate-Orange Energy Balls (see page 64)

Spending a Sunday morning making your snacks for the week can really add something extra to your meals and with every one of these lunches; the humble carrot takes on multiple personalities. The Basic Granola is another incredibly customizable recipe. Here it's used for 4 out of the 5 days but by serving it with all sorts of bits and pieces, you get a totally different brekkie every day. A little forethought and planning can make all the difference and by being efficient with your shopping it will not only save you loads of time in the long run but also save you some money!

WEDNESDAY	THURSDAY	FRIDAY
Raspberry Chia Seed Jar (see page 22)	Basic Granola (see page 14)	Cherry Coconut Granola Jar (see page 16)
Winter Warmer Soup (see page 39) with sprinkling of Spicy Crunchy Chickpeas (see page 60) on top or as an afternoon snack	Giant Couscous and Heritage Carrot Salad Jar (see page 40) Nut Butter and Fruit Crisps (see page 63)	Winter Warmer Soup (see page 39) with sprinkling of Spicy Crunchy Chickpeas (see page 60) on top or as an afternoon snack

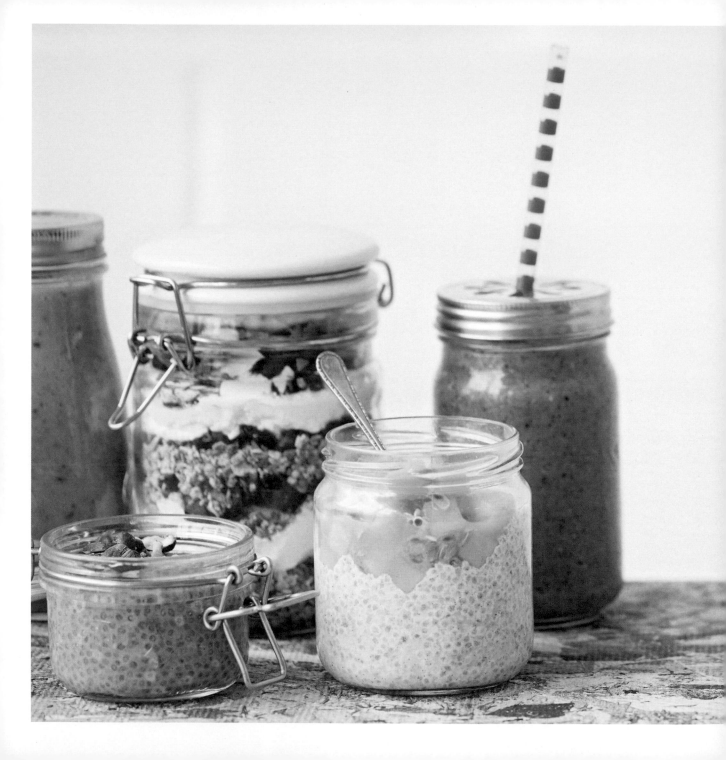

BREAKFASTS

Breakfast is often the meal we skip the most due to rushing around in the morning, trying to get out of the door and not thinking about sitting down for ten minutes when we'd rather have that time in bed. Preparing jars the night before or assembling a quick last-minute jar for on the road makes fitting breakfast in doable. In this chapter there is a mix of speedy weekday recipes as well as some more long weekend-type jars to give you lots of choice about how you kick-start your day.

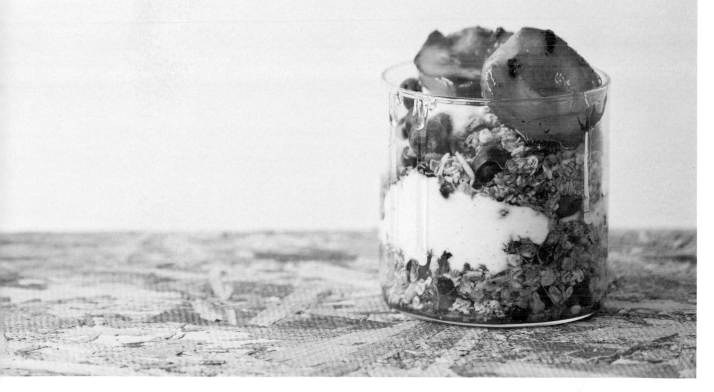

COCONUT & CHIA OVERNIGHT OATS

INGREDIENTS

Makes 1 x 500ml/18fl oz jar
Keeps: 2 days

2 tbsp coconut yogurt
150ml/5fl oz/⅔ cup milk
    (I used a coconut rice blend)
80g/3oz/generous ¾ cup
    rolled oats
2 tbsp chia seeds
2 tbsp desiccated
    (dry unsweetened
    shredded) coconut
½ tsp vanilla bean paste
pinch of salt
2 tbsp honey, plus extra to serve
assorted berries; strawberries,
    raspberries, blueberries,
    to serve

I'm a big fan of classic porridge and so was a little unsure as to how I would feel about cold oats, but these are delicious! I have eaten them straight from the refrigerator on the bus to work and have also warmed them up – both are equally yummy. Frozen berries are a great alternative to fresh in the colder months – they thaw slightly en route for an extra texture combo.

The night before or at least 5 hours before you want to eat the oats, mix all the ingredients, except the berries, together in a large bowl. Pop them all into your jar, pop the lid on and leave overnight in the refrigerator.

When ready to eat, fill your jar to the top with berries and drizzle over some extra honey.

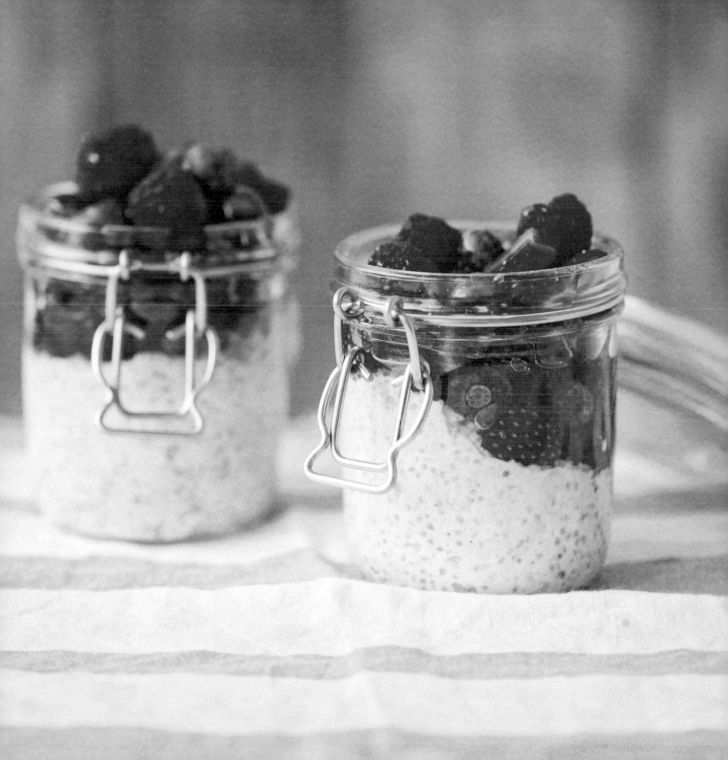

BASIC GRANOLA

INGREDIENTS

Makes 1 litre/35fl oz jar
Keeps: Up to 4 weeks

200g/7oz/⅔ cup maple syrup
4 tbsp honey
40g/1¼oz/scant ¼ cup coconut
  oil, melted
450g/1lb/4¾ cups rolled jumbo
  oats
100g/3½oz/¾ cup pumpkin
  seeds
100g/3½oz/¾ cup sunflower
  seeds
2 tbsp flaxseeds
2 tbsp sesame seeds

Optional extras
250g/9oz/2 cups nuts, such as
  almonds, pecans and walnuts
250g/9oz/1½ cups dried fruit,
  such as apricots, cherries,
  banana chips and sultanas
  (golden raisins)

Granola is such a versatile breakfast – you can add anything you like to a batch and create so many different flavours. My favourites are the large crunchy clusters so when you are mixing it halfway through baking, don't be too heavy handed – a gentle smoothing round with a wooden spoon will be all it needs to stop it catching. This basic recipe leaves the creativity up to you and I will be showing you three of my favourite ways to liven up your jars (see pages 15-19).

Preheat the oven to 170°C/325°F/Gas mark 3.

Warm the maple syrup, honey and coconut oil together in a pan to make them easier to mix with the other granola ingredients.

Stir the oats and seeds together in a large bowl, stir in the maple syrup mix, then add the nuts, if using, and stir to make sure everything is evenly coated.

Spread the mixture out on 1–2 baking trays and bake in the hot oven for 20-30 minutes, stirring the mixture occasionally so it bakes evenly.

Leave the granola to cool on the trays to crisp up. Chop up the dried fruit, if using, and add as your pour into an airtight 1 litre/35fl oz jar.

APPLE CRUMBLE GRANOLA

INGREDIENTS

Makes 1 x 500ml/18fl oz jar
Keeps: 3 days (without yogurt)

2 eating apples, cored and
   chopped
½ tsp each of ground cinnamon,
   nutmeg and ginger
2 tbsp honey or maple syrup
grated zest and juice of 1 lemon
5 heaped tbsp Greek yogurt
handful of Basic Granola made
   with sultanas (golden raisins)
   and pecans (see page 14)

When the nights draw in, there's something comforting about apple crumble so what better way to start your day than with a breakfast version. This quick and easy apple compote can be made a day ahead or served hot piled on top of your yogurt and granola. If the variety of apple you would use is naturally quite sweet, omit the honey or maple syrup, but it does add a rounded flavour, so test as you go and see what you like.

Place the apples in a pan with the spices, honey or maple syrup and the lemon zest and juice. Cook over a low heat until the apples are soft and your kitchen smells heavenly. Add a drop of water if the apples look too dry.

Pop some Greek yogurt into your jar, then add a layer of apple compote. Continue with the layers until you reach the top and finish with a thick layer of granola, just before you leave the house. This ensures you still have some lovely crunchy bits, even if you can't eat it straightaway.

CHERRY COCONUT GRANOLA JAR

INGREDIENTS

Makes 1 x 500ml/18fl oz jar
Keeps: 3 days (without yogurt)

5–8 tbsp coconut yogurt
2 tbsp coconut shavings
handful of Basic Granola made
    with dried cherries and
    almonds (see page 14)
handful of fresh cherries or
    about 10 canned cherries,
    pitted

Cherry and coconut is an awesome combo. When cherries are at their best there really is no better fruit. Canned cherries don't quite pack the same punch but are a great alternative during winter. I sometimes reduce the juice from the can and add it as an extra drizzle on top - seriously worth it. Coconut yogurt is relatively new to hit the supermarkets but it is there hiding away with the soya milks, etc. There are also tutorials online about how to make your own. Dried cherries here make all the difference to the sweetness; they are a bit of an investment but worth it. Lots of them are resoaked in apple juice, but don't let this put you off, as they're even tastier.

Pop some coconut yogurt into your jar, followed by the cherries.

Toast the coconut shavings in a dry frying pan (skillet) over a medium heat until they are starting to turn golden brown - keep them moving around to stop them burning. Leave to cool and crisp up.

Top the jar with the granola, then scatter over the coconut shavings. The cherries should stop the granola going soggy while you travel (if you are going for a multi-layered jar make sure a cherry layer surrounds the granola), but mix it up well when you are ready to eat to make sure you get everything on your spoon.

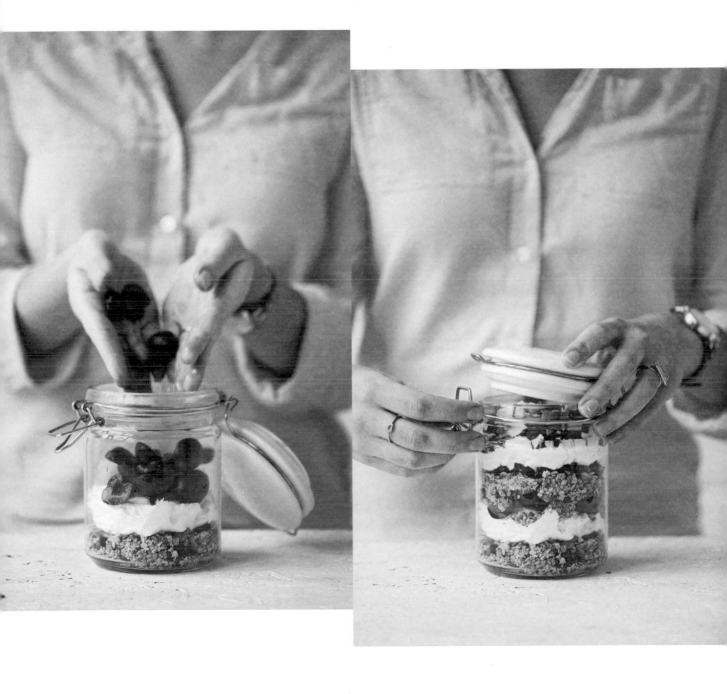

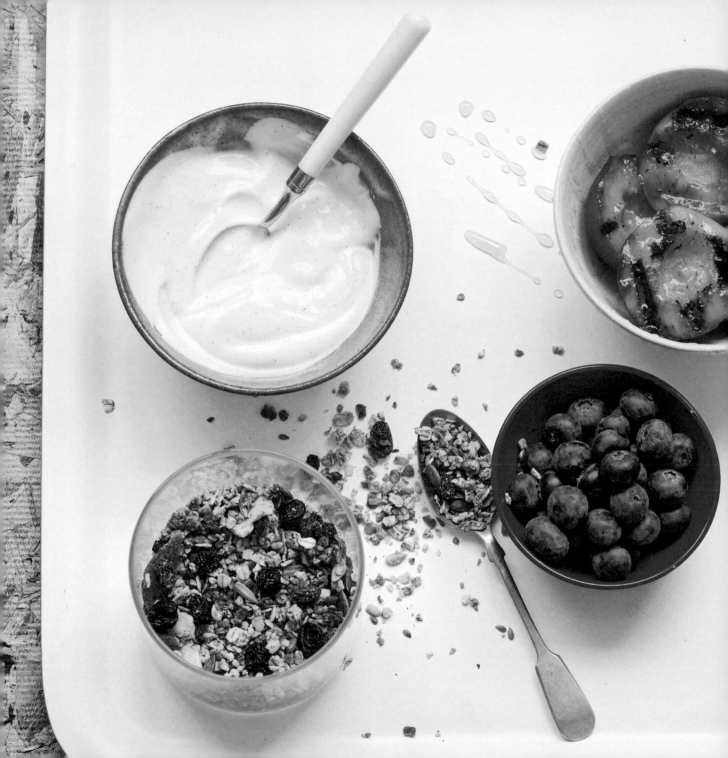

GRILLED STONE FRUIT JAR WITH VANILLA AND ALMONDS

INGREDIENTS

Makes 1 x 500ml/18fl oz jar
Keeps: 3 days (without yogurt)

handful of Basic Granola made
    with whole almonds and dried
    blueberries (see page 14)
1 nectarine or persimmon
1 tbsp maple syrup (optional)
5 heaped tbsp plain yogurt
1 tsp vanilla bean paste
handful of blueberries
1 tbsp coconut almond butter
    (optional)
extra whole almonds, to serve
    (optional)

Summer gives us wonderful stone fruits and any of them are wonderful when grilled. When autumn (fall) arrives, persimmons (sometimes called kaki fruit) are a lovely alternative, many markets have them spilling out of their displays. There are so many nut butters available, so make sure you find one without any palm oil and the fewest ingredients possible – it should just be nuts and a couple of other bits. My favourite at the moment is Pip & Nut's Coconut Almond Butter – swirled through this jar it just works so well. You could also have a go at making your own (see page 63).

When making the granola according to the instructions on page 14 add lots of extra almonds before baking and stir through the dried blueberries after baking.

For the grilled stone fruit, start by slicing them into wedges and patting dry with kitchen paper. Heat a griddle pan and lay the fruit across it – don't touch for 2–3 minutes to ensure that the fruit has some lovely char lines over it. Flip over when they are golden and cook the other side for a further 2 minutes. Pop the fruit into a bowl and coat in the maple syrup, if using.

Whisk the yogurt with the vanilla bean paste, then place it into the bottom of your jar. Add the chargrilled fruit followed by the blueberries and finish with the granola, some nut butter and extra almonds, if you like.

BERRY QUINOA PORRIDGE

INGREDIENTS

Makes 1 x 500ml/18fl oz jar
Keeps: 2–3 days

60g/21/4oz/⅓ cup quinoa,
  rinsed
280ml/10fl oz/scant 1¼ cups
  milk (coconut, almond, cow's)
½ cinnamon stick
1 tsp vanilla bean paste or
  extract
1 tbsp maple syrup
pinch of salt
frozen berries (optional), to serve

There are so many awesome grains out there and using them for alternatives at breakfast is such a good way of trying out something new. Quinoa, in particular, has a super-high protein content and is full of fibre. Being wheat-free it is also suitable for people following a gluten-free diet, so serving a big steaming bowl of this on a Sunday morning is always well received. Mix up your milks when making it and find your favourite - mine is coconut. It is a great dairy-free alternative that adds bags of flavour and tastes utterly delicious with whatever else you pile on top.

Place the rinsed quinoa in a pan over a low heat and add 200ml/7fl oz/scant 1 cup of the milk, the cinnamon stick and vanilla. Cover with a lid and cook for 8–10 minutes until most of the liquid has been absorbed. Be very careful as it can easily boil over. Add the remaining milk, the maple syrup and salt and stir gently until the porridge has thickened to your liking. Take off the heat and remove and discard the cinnamon stick. Pop the porridge into your jar and top with anything you like. I love adding a handful of frozen berries just before I leave the house as they thaw beautifully when I reheat the porridge at work.

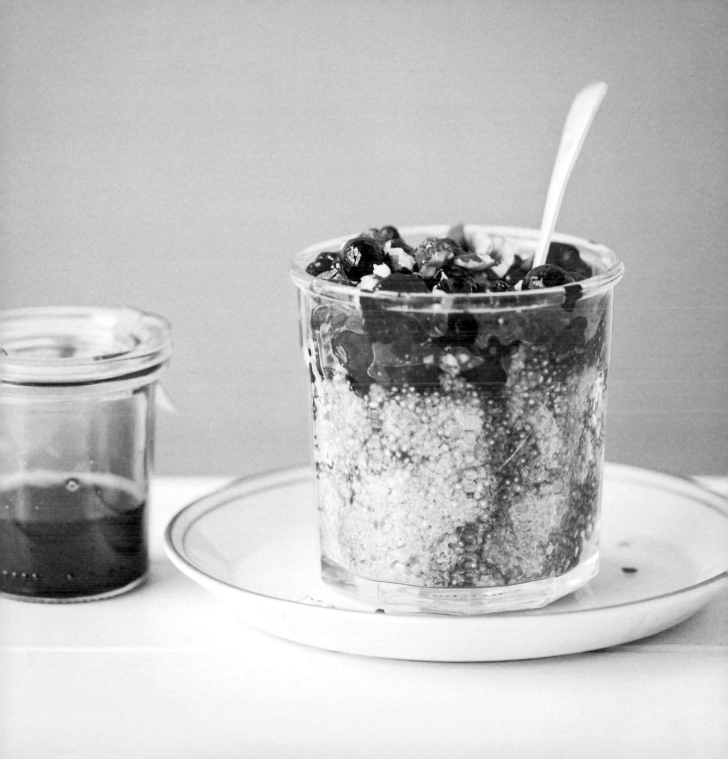

CHIA SEED JARS

INGREDIENTS

Each recipe makes 1 x 500ml/
   18fl oz jar
Keeps: 3–4 days

Chia seed pudding can have a bad reputation, as it is sometimes thought of as being slimy, but the creaminess of this pudding takes that away entirely. Chia seeds are some of the healthiest little dudes out there: they are packed with fibre and protein and loads of great vitamins and antioxidants too – all good stuff. All three of these variations are totally different so try them all and see which one is your favourite. Any berry can be used instead of raspberries, so if strawberries are crying your name, then go for it.

RASPBERRY CHIA SEED JAR

INGREDIENTS

½ punnet of raspberries (about
   100g/3½oz/1 cup)
200ml/7fl oz/scant 1 cup almond
   milk
1 tbsp honey
2½ tbsp chia seeds
whole almonds, crushed,
   to serve

Set aside a few rasberries for serving, then whizz the remaining raspberries with the milk and honey in a blender or food processor until smooth. Pour into your jar and add the chia seeds. Pop the lid on and give a quick shake. Leave the jar overnight in the refrigerator.

The next morning, top the pudding with some crushed almonds and the reserved raspberries, and you are good to go!

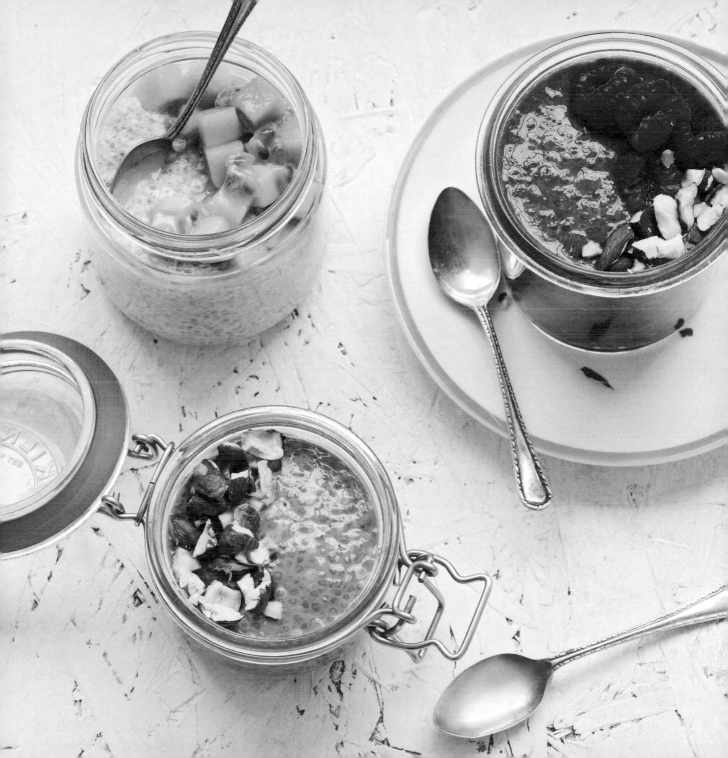

TROPICAL CHIA SEED JAR

INGREDIENTS

150ml/5fl oz/⅔ cup coconut milk
50g/1¾oz/3½ tbsp coconut or plain yogurt
2½ tbsp chia seeds
1 tsp maple syrup
½ tsp vanilla bean paste or extract
1 tbsp desiccated (dry unsweetened shredded) coconut
½ mango, diced
1 passion fruit

Stir the milk, yogurt, chia seeds, maple syrup, vanilla and desiccated coconut together in a bowl until well combined.

Mix the mango and passion fruit seeds together in a separate bowl, then leave both overnight in the refrigerator, stirring the chia pudding a couple of times to ensure that it doesn't clump together.

The next morning, layer up the chia pudding and fruit in your jar, finishing with the fruit on top.

MATCHA CHIA SEED JAR

INGREDIENTS

150ml/5fl oz/⅔ cup hazelnut
   milk
1 tbsp honey
½ tsp matcha tea (Japanese
   green tea powder)
pinch of salt
2½ tbsp chia seeds
toasted hazelnuts, to serve

Place the milk, honey, matcha tea and salt in your jar, pop the lid on and shake very well to make sure that the matcha blends well with the ingredients. If there are still lumps use a small whisk to whisk the mixture to a smooth green paste.

Add the chia seeds, pop the lid on again and shake. Leave the jar overnight in the refrigerator, shaking the pudding after 20 minutes or so to make sure the chia seeds aren't sticking together.

The next morning, top with the toasted hazelnuts and enjoy!

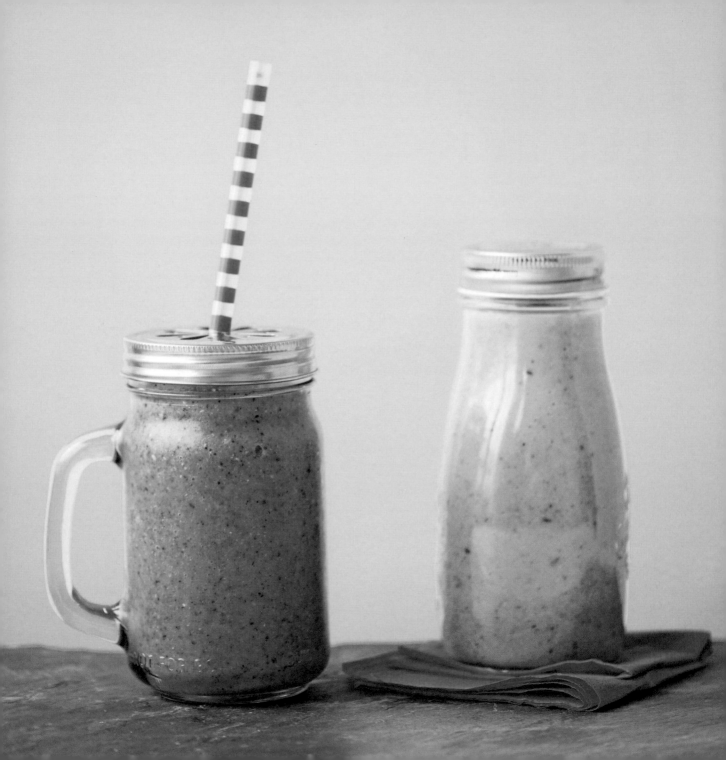

BANANA BERRY COCONUT SMOOTHIE

INGREDIENTS

Makes 1 x 500ml/18fl oz jar
Keeps: 1–2 days

200ml/7fl oz/scant 1 cup
    coconut milk
1 tsp coconut oil
1 tsp vanilla bean paste
1 banana, frozen
handful of frozen mixed berries
2 tsp honey, to taste

Coconut oil has a whole host of health benefits and adding a teaspoon to a smoothie is an easy way to get it into your diet. Coconut milk is also a great dairy-free alternative and adds an awesome flavour to the berries and banana. To have this all year round, I tend to keep those mixed frozen berry bags in the freezer - they also chill the smoothie down very well. If using fresh fruit, just add a small handful of ice.

Pop everything into a blender and pulse a few times to get it started. Scrape down the sides and have a quick taste then blend continuously until smooth. Add the honey, if you like a slightly sweeter smoothie, then pour into your jar. Leave in the fridge until serving.

SUPER GREEN SUPER SMOOTHIE

INGREDIENTS

Makes 1 x 500ml/18fl oz jar
Keeps: 1–2 days

1 large handful of spinach
½ pineapple, chopped
1 peach, pitted
grated zest and juice of 1 lime
1 banana, chopped and frozen
¼ cucumber, chopped
2 tbsp yogurt (plain, coconut,
    etc.)
100ml/3½fl oz/scant ½ cup
    almond milk
few mint sprigs
ice cubes (optional)

Some green smoothies have a tendency to taste rather savoury and nothing but 'green', but I prefer a sweeter taste. Packing this one full of fruit takes the edge off the spinach and you have a lovely hit of 'green'. Any bananas that are looking a little worse for wear are perfect for this one; keep a few chopped up in the freezer as they add so much to the texture of any smoothie, but if you don't have any frozen to hand, a normal one will do.

Pop everything into a blender and pulse to get it started. Push the spinach down and stir well. Continue to blend until smooth, adding a small handful of ice to chill it down if you're not using a frozen banana. When smooth, pour into your jar, pop the lid on and chill in the refrigerator until you are ready to get your boost!

CRANBERRY AND ALMOND BIRCHER MUESLI

INGREDIENTS

Makes 1 x 500ml/18fl oz jar
Keeps: 2 days (without milk and
    yogurt)

The night before
40g/1½oz/scant ½ cup rolled
    jumbo oats
20g/¾oz/scant ¼ cup dried
    cranberries
100ml/3½fl oz/scant ½ cup
    apple juice

The next morning
1 eating apple, coarsely grated
50ml/2fl oz/3½ tbsp almond milk

To serve
plain yogurt
flaked (slivered) almonds
honey

Bircher muesli seems to have fallen off the radar recently, but it is one of my absolute favourite things to start my day. Anything fresh and fruity but still has that creaminess we love in oats is always a good thing and this is no exception. I use dried cranberries as the tang of them with the apple make a delicious version for me, but try other variations, such as adding a teaspoon of cinnamon and using sultanas (golden raisins) or adding some desiccated (dry unsweetened shredded) coconut to the overnight mix for a tropical twist.

The night before, stir the oats, cranberries and apple juice together in your jar. Pop the lid on and place in the refrigerator to soak overnight.

The next morning, add the grated apple to the jar and stir through the almond milk until combined. To serve, add a dollop of yogurt, a sprinkling of flaked (slivered) almonds and a drizzle of honey.

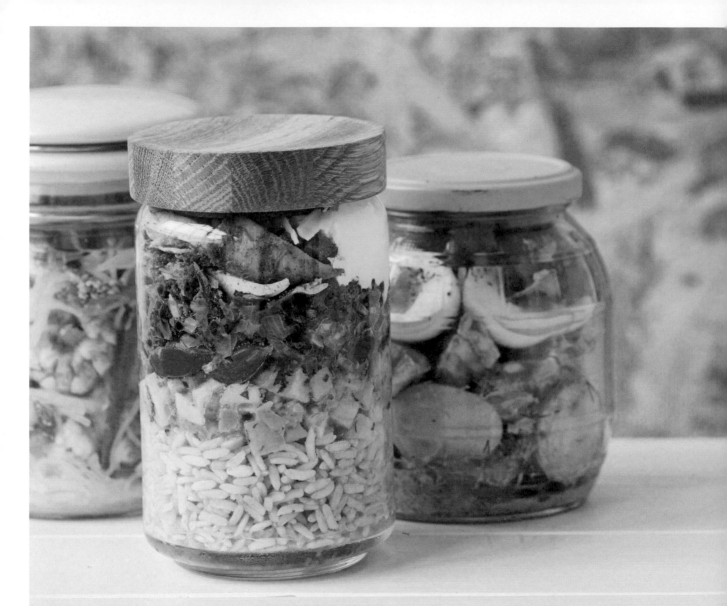

MAIN MEALS

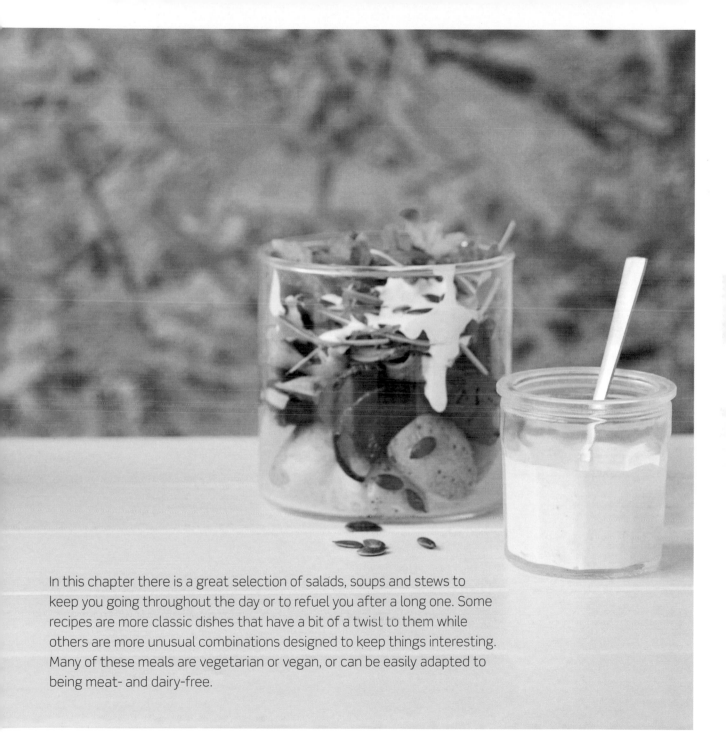

In this chapter there is a great selection of salads, soups and stews to keep you going throughout the day or to refuel you after a long one. Some recipes are more classic dishes that have a bit of a twist to them while others are more unusual combinations designed to keep things interesting. Many of these meals are vegetarian or vegan, or can be easily adapted to being meat- and dairy-free.

SUSHI JAR

INGREDIENTS

Makes 1 x 700ml/25fl oz jar
Keeps: 3 days

150g/5¼oz/¾ cup sushi rice
200ml/7fl oz/scant 1 cup water
2 tbsp rice vinegar
1 tsp salt
1 tsp palm sugar or use brown
    sugar
¼ cucumber
1 carrot
½ avocado
juice of ½ lime
smoked salmon or tofu (optional)
1 nori sheet
soy sauce, to taste
wasabi, to taste
pickled ginger, to taste
black sesame seeds, for
    sprinkling

There are few things I could eat forever but sushi has to be one of them. If I had the time to make it every day I would love to. This is a super-quick way of getting all the best bits but without the tricky and time-consuming rolling. Most large supermarkets have a great Asian foods section where you can find everything you need to make great sushi jars. I've used the California roll as an inspiration, however, using totally unauthentic smoked salmon. It tastes great and is far cheaper than sushi-grade salmon, as well as being readily available so for me, what's not to love?

Thoroughly rinse the rice in a sieve (strainer) until the water runs clear, then place in a pan with the water and heat over a low heat. When bubbling, cover with a lid and leave for 6–8 minutes until the water has been absorbed. Mix the vinegar, salt and sugar together in a bowl until the salt and sugar have dissolved. (You can always pop it in the microwave for 10 seconds to help it along.) When the rice is done, using a wooden spoon, scrape the rice into a bowl and add the rice vinegar seasoning. Leave to cool at room temperature, then store in the refrigerator until ready to use.

To make your sushi jar, chop the cucumber and carrot into matchsticks. Dice the avocado and toss in the lime juice to avoid discoloration. Get your protein ready, if using, and slice the nori sheet into bite-sized squares for easy eating.

Layer up! I start with a layer of nori bits and rice followed by a drizzle of soy sauce, a splodge of wasabi and some pickled ginger. Then I add a few bits of each vegetable and some lovely salmon. Throughout I sprinkle a few black sesame seeds and keep layering until I reach the top. You can, of course, finish with more wasabi and ginger, if you like. I finish with a few more layers of nori to keep it crisp.

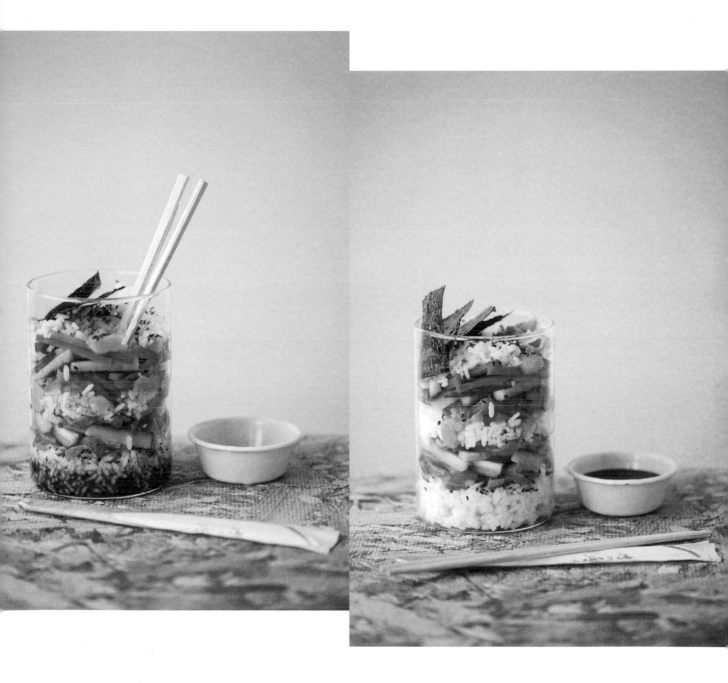

VIETNAMESE-INSPIRED NOODLE SALAD

INGREDIENTS

Makes 1 x 700ml/25fl oz jar
Keeps: 2 days

For the dressing
1 garlic clove, very finely chopped
5cm/2in piece of fresh ginger, peeled and very finely chopped
1 red chilli, finely sliced
1 tbsp fish sauce (omit for vegan version)
grated zest and juice of 1 lime
1 tbsp palm sugar or use brown sugar
1 tbsp groundnut (peanut) oil or use any flavourless oil
½ tsp sesame oil

For the salad
100g/3½oz raw prawns (shrimp) or tofu
50g/1¾oz noodles (glass noodles are awesome but rice vermicelli also works well)
50g/1¾oz sugar snap peas, halved
1 carrot, cut into matchsticks
½ courgette (zucchini), spiralised or cut into matchsticks
2 spring onions (scallions), finely sliced
small handful of beansprouts
small bunch of coriander (cilantro), chopped
2 tbsp sesame seeds, toasted

This salad packs a proper punch and is perfect for both a fresh summer's lunch and a much needed brightening during winter. Cut everything as fine as you can to make sure it is coated in the lovely dressing. This keeps particularly well thanks to the dressing, so it's perfect to double up for a couple of days' worth of lunches. I love the freshness of peas and prawns here but you can easily switch it for some marinated tofu to make it vegan, if you like!

Start by putting all the dressing ingredients into a jar, covering with the lid and shaking well. Pour 1 tbsp over the prawns to allow them to start marinating.

Cook the noodles by putting them into a heatproof bowl and pouring boiling water over them. Leave to stand while you prepare all the veg. They should still have a bit of bite to them so check them every so often, then drain and separate.

Put all the salad ingredients, except the prawns and sesame seeds, into your jar, pop the lid on and shake well to mix everything up.

Fry the marinated prawns in a pan until they are just pink, if using, then add them to the jar. Or add the tofu. Pour over the remaining dressing, sprinkle with the toasted sesame seeds and chill in the refrigerator until ready to eat.

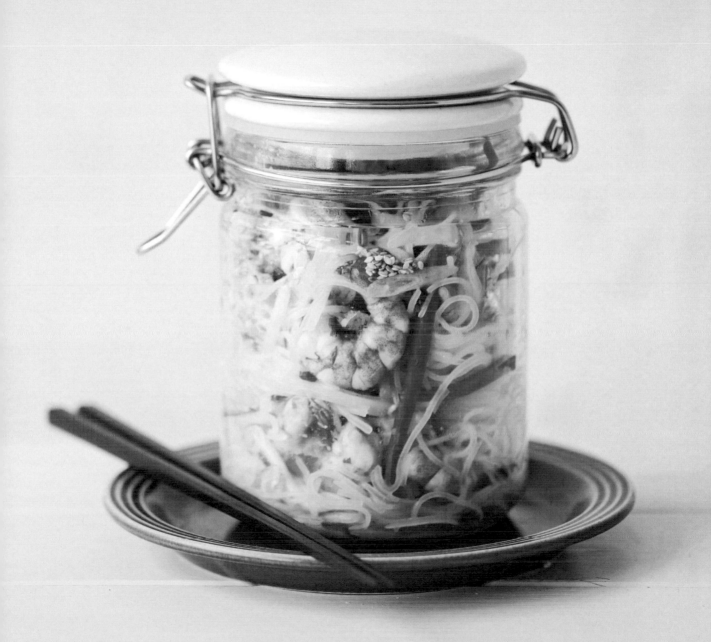

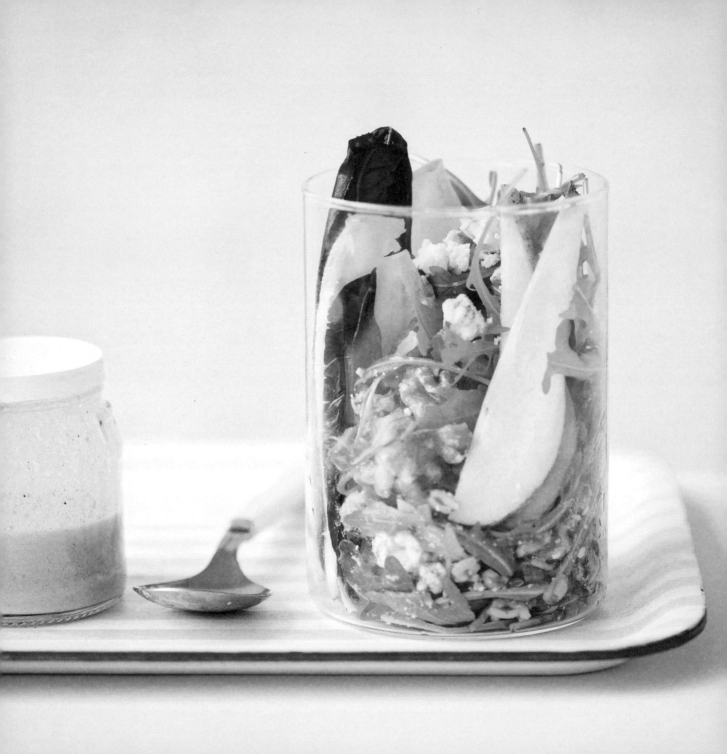

PEAR, STILTON AND WALNUT SALAD JAR

INGREDIENTS

Makes 1 x 700ml/25fl oz jar
Keeps: 4 days (without dressing)

For the dressing
2 tbsp walnut oil
juice of ½ lemon
2 tsp Dijon mustard
1 tsp white wine vinegar

For the salad
100g/3½oz spelt berries
300ml/10fl oz/1¼ cups hot
   water or stock
1 endive bulb
large handful of rocket (arugula)
50g/1¾oz/1 cup walnut halves
100g/3½oz Stilton
3 prosciutto slices (optional)
1 pear, sliced and dressed in a
   squeeze of lemon to prevent
   browning

There are many perfect triplets in the world and this is certainly one of them. It's such a simple salad and can be totally personalised with any extra veg you have to boost it if you wish. Spelt is the slightly more nutritious cousin of wheat. It adds bulk to this otherwise light offering and can easily be changed to a gluten-free 'grain', such as quinoa, if you prefer. If making the day before, leave your dressing in its own jar and drizzle over just as you are eating – this stops the leaves wilting and gives your dressing a little longer to develop in flavour – never a bad thing.

Soak the spelt berries for the salad overnight.

The next day, make the dressing. Pop everything into a small jar, cover with the lid and shake to combine. Chill in the refrigerator until ready to serve.

To cook the spelt berries, rinse them in clean water and drain. Place in a pan with the hot water or stock. Cover with a lid and simmer over a low heat for 45 minutes, or until the spelt berries are soft.

Prepare the salad by slicing the endive into long pieces and tossing through with the rocket. Slice your pear lengthways and toss in lemon juice to keep it fresh.

Next, toast the walnuts in a dry frying pan (skillet) over a low heat to release all the gorgeous oils. Keep them moving so they don't catch, and remove when you can smell their lovely nutty flavour.

In a large bowl fold together your spelt, rocket, walnut and Stilton. Add to the jar with the endive leaves and sliced pear, finishing with the prosciutto torn into long strips, if using. Drizzle over the dressing when you're ready to eat, then pop on the lid and shake gently so everything is coated in the dressing.

POMEGRANATE PILAF

INGREDIENTS

Makes 1 x 700ml/25fl oz jar
Keeps: 3 days

1 tbsp coconut oil
½ tsp cumin seeds
½ tsp sumac
½ tsp ground coriander
3 cardamom pods, lightly
   crushed
2 cloves
1 small white onion, diced
1 garlic clove, very finely
   chopped
1 carrot, diced
1 bay leaf, fresh or dried
50g/1¾oz/scant ½ cup cashew
   nuts
1 tbsp pomegranate ketchup,
   such as Aphrodite's
100g/3½oz/½ cup brown short-
   grain rice, rinsed
900ml/1½ pints/3½ cups
   vegetable stock
½ pomegranate, seeds removed
small handful of flat-leaf parsley,
   chopped
50g/1¾oz feta cheese, (optional)

A pilaf is such a lovely comforting thing and this one with the warm sweetness of pomegranate and spices, comforts in just the right amounts. The seeds give a burst of juicy freshness and the cashews cook down to a strikingly different texture from normal. Rice is an awesome lunch option – full of fibre and vitamins to keep you going all afternoon. I love using brown short-grain rice for its nutty taste but any rice variety will do. This jar is also delicious as a side dish for two so keep that in mind if you fall in love with it.

Heat the oil in a large pan and add all the spices. Keep them moving around the pan quickly for about 15–20 seconds, then add the onion, garlic and carrot and stir to coat in the spices. Add the bay leaf and cashews and cook for 2 minutes. Add the pomegranate ketchup, then add the rice. Add 300ml/10fl oz/1¼ cups of the stock and stir. Cover with a lid and cook for about 10 minutes. Check the rice every now and then and add more stock as necessary until it starts to look tender. Cook for a total of about 30 minutes (slightly less if using white rice).

When the rice is done, remove and discard the bay leaf, fluff up the rice with a fork and stir through the pomegranate seeds. Scatter the parsley and cheese over the top, if using. This is delicious both hot and cold but beware of the cloves and cardamom pods.

WINTER WARMER SOUP

INGREDIENTS

Makes 2 x 500ml/18fl oz jars
Keeps: 5 days

½ small butternut squash,
  deseeded (see Top Tip below)
1 parsnip
1 carrot
1 red (bell) pepper
1 celery stick
1 tbsp coconut or olive oil
1 tsp dried chilli flakes (hot red
  pepper flakes)
1 tsp cumin seeds
1 tsp dried thyme
sea salt and freshly ground black
  pepper
1 litre/1¾ pints/4 cups vegetable
  stock
400ml/14fl oz can coconut milk

TOP TIP!
Roast the butternut squash
seeds with some oil and salt and
serve those on top as a crunchy
addition!

Autumn (fall) is without doubt, my favourite season. Everything seems to glow with gorgeous golds and robust reds and root vegetables really come to the fore. This is a soup full of flavour with gentle spices giving you that warm-from-the-inside-out feeling that's so comforting when it's chilly outside. This is a thick soup to fill me up but if you like a looser texture, just add some more stock when you are blending the mixture. Keep tasting throughout and add more salt and pepper than you think you need, as it mellows out as it chills. You need about 500–600g/1lb 2oz–1¼lb of any root veg you have.

Preheat the oven to 170°C/325°F/Gas mark 3.

Chop all the vegetables into even-sized pieces – leave the skins on to enhance the flavour. Place the vegetables in a roasting tin, add the oil, spices, thyme and seasoning and toss together until coated. Roast in the hot oven for about 30 minutes, or until cooked through and slightly brown on the edges.

Transfer the vegetables to a large pan over a low heat and add the stock and coconut milk. Cook for a further 20–30 minutes, adding more salt and pepper as needed. Blend the mixture with a stick blender to the consistency that you like, then pour into your jars.

Eat straight away or leave to cool and then refrigerate before reheating (see page 7 for tips).

GIANT COUSCOUS AND HERITAGE CARROT SALAD JAR

INGREDIENTS

Makes 1 x 700ml/25fl oz jar
Keeps: 4 days (without dressing)

300ml/10fl oz/1¼ cups
    vegetable stock
100g/3½oz/½ cup dried giant
    wholewheat couscous
small handful of flat-leaf parsley,
    chopped
250g/9oz heritage carrots (I
    particularly love purple ones)
few thyme sprigs, leaves picked
½ tsp cumin seeds
grated zest of 1 orange
3 tbsp olive oil
3 tbsp plain yogurt
grated zest and juice of ½ lemon
1 garlic clove, very finely
    chopped
sea salt and freshly ground black
    pepper
small handful of rocket (arugula)
30g/1oz/scant ¼ cup golden
    sultanas (golden raisins)

Bigger is better when it comes to couscous – giant couscous soaks up so much more flavour than their tiny counterparts. They need slightly more attention, however, but cooking on the hob (stove top) with stock doesn't take too long. With a creamy yogurt dressing like this one, it's important to keep it separate until serving as the couscous will definitely absorb it all – losing all that awesome contrast of cool tangy yogurt and sweet carroty goodness. You can keep it in a smaller jar or just use the rocket as a barrier between the two.

Preheat the oven to 160°C/325°F/Gas mark 3.

Bring the stock to the boil in a pan, then add the couscous. Cover with a lid, reduce the heat and simmer for about 6 minutes, or until the couscous is soft but still with a bite. Remove from the heat and leave to cool. When the couscous is cool, fold through the chopped parsley, then set aside in the pan.

While the couscous is cooling, cut the carrots into long sticks and toss in the thyme, cumin, orange zest and 2 tbsp olive oil. Place them on a baking tray and roast in the hot oven for 20–30 minutes until tender. When done, stir the roasted carrots into the couscous with all the roasting juices.

To make the dressing, mix the yogurt, lemon, remaining olive oil and garlic with some seasoning in a small jar and keep refrigerated until serving – just don't forget it in the morning!

Start filling your jar with the couscous and carrots, followed by the rocket and sultanas. Add the dressing in lovely dollops and mix it up a bit for maximum flavour.

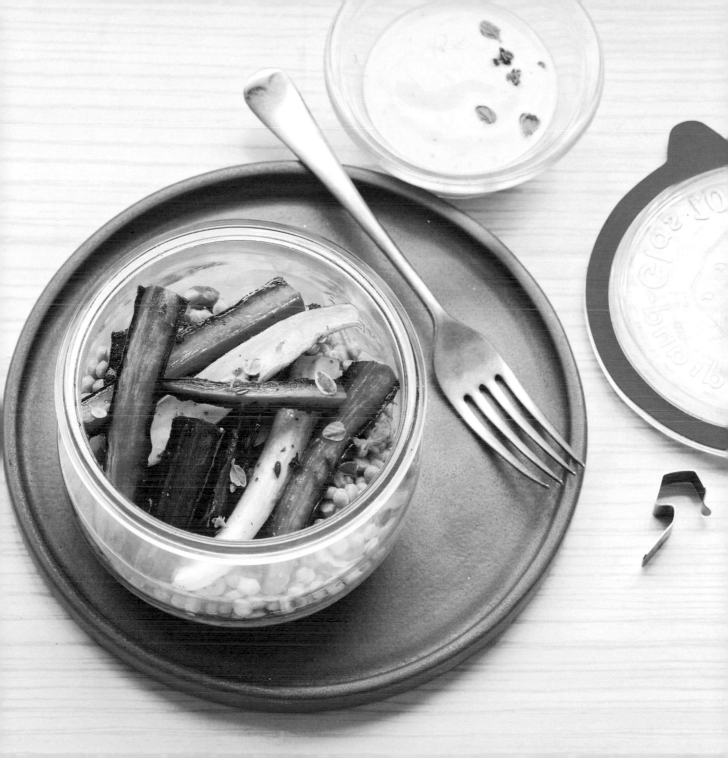

HOT SMOKED SALMON AND WATERCRESS SALAD WITH LEMON CAPER DRESSING

INGREDIENTS

Makes 1 x 700ml/25fl oz jar
Keeps: 3–4 days

5–6 baby potatoes, halved
2 eggs
1 tbsp capers, chopped
few dill sprigs
grated zest and juice of ½ lemon
1 tbsp olive oil
½ tsp each salt and freshly
    ground black pepper
½ tsp Dijon mustard
1 hot smoked salmon fillet,
    broken into large flakes
½ bunch of watercress

This is a super-simple recipe – more of a put together than anything else! If you are short on time this is perfect as it takes just the time of boiling the potatoes. This recipe can be kept in the refrigerator for up to four days and can be easily warmed in the oven or microwave (minus the watercress), so it's a great one to prep for the week if you fancy something fresh but comforting. The soft-boiled eggs add a wonderful richness, which works very well with the sharpness of the dressing.

Cook the potatoes in a pan of boiling water for 10–12 minutes - test them with a knife and if it goes in cleanly with no resistance, they are done. Remove them with a slotted spoon and gently lower the eggs into the water and set a timer for 6 minutes. As soon as the eggs are done, run them under cold running water so they are easier to peel. Peel them both and set aside.

To make the dressing, put the capers, dill, lemon zest and juice, olive oil, salt and pepper and mustard into a small jar, pop the lid on and shake well.

Start filling your jar with the hot smoked salmon, then add the soft-boiled eggs and potatoes. Drizzle in half the dressing, then add the watercress and the remaining dressing. If you want to heat it up, remove the watercress gently and set aside while the jar is warming. Put it back in and serve.

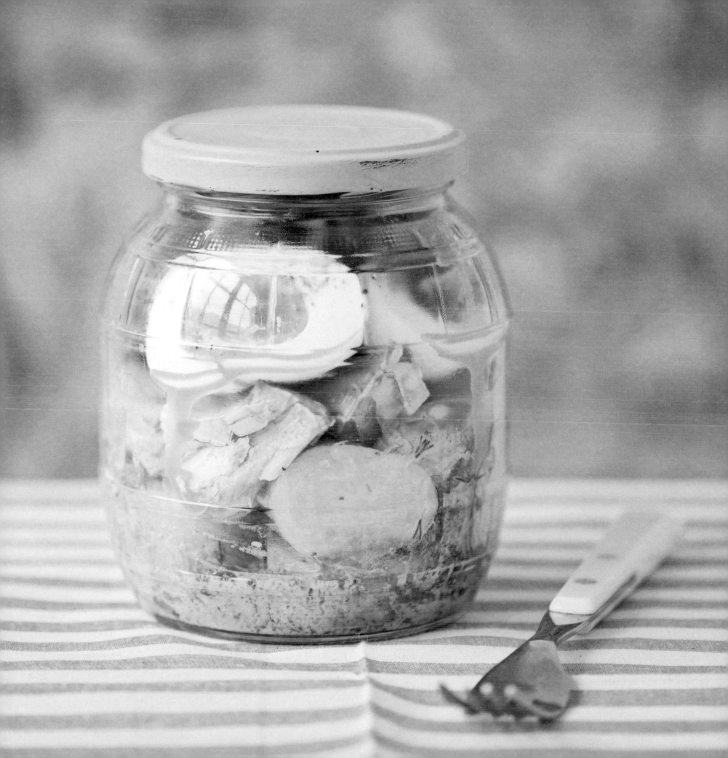

BURRITO JAR

INGREDIENTS

Makes 1 x 700ml/25fl oz jar
Keeps: 3 days (without
   guacamole)

1 boneless and skinless chicken
   thigh or your favourite veg
1 tsp ground cumin
1 tsp paprika
2 tbsp olive oil
175g/6oz/scant 1 cup brown
rice, cooked and cooled (or ½
   pack of microwave rice)
3–4 tbsp sour cream
50g/1¾oz/½ cup Cheddar
   cheese, grated

For the salsa
handful of cherry tomatoes,
   chopped
large pinch of sea salt
½ red onion, finely diced
½ red chilli (chile), finely chopped
grated zest of 1 lime
1 tsp white wine vinegar
1 tbsp olive oil

For the guacamole
½ avocado
juice of 1 lime
small handful of coriander
   (cilantro), stalks reserved for
   the black beans
large pinch of sea salt
freshly ground black pepper
   (optional)

Making your own burrito means you get all the best bits (and don't pay extra for the guac, am I right?) You can also control the spice levels in the salsa to be as mild or as hot as you like. Don't forget the sour cream and cheese on top – it seems excessive but it really does bring the whole jar together and adds a necessary coolness and richness. If you have the time, marinate your chicken or extra veg overnight in the rub, but if you are pushed for time and can manage only 15 minutes it's still delicious. If you can, make your guacamole the night before you eat it - any longer and despite the lime juice, it will start to turn brown. Keep the avocado stone in the guacamole overnight as this can limit its bronzing.

Start by making the salsa and guacamole. To make the salsa, mix the chopped tomatoes and salt together in a bowl, then leave for a few minutes to draw out some awesome flavour. Add the remaining ingredients and stir. Leave at room temperature until serving if making on the day or in the fridge overnight. For the guacamole, mash everything together in a bowl, adding a twist of pepper, if you wish. Set aside.

Marinate the chicken or chosen vegetable in the cumin, paprika and olive oil for at least 15 minutes, or preferably overnight in the refrigerator.

For the black beans, heat a glug of olive oil in a pan over a low heat, add the white onion, spring onions, coriander stalks and garlic and cook gently until softened. Add the black beans and cook until they are warmed through and slightly broken down.

For the black beans

1 tbsp olive oil

1 small white onion, finely diced

2 spring onions (scallions), chopped

coriander (cilantro) stalks, chopped (from the guacamole)

1 garlic clove, finely chopped

½ can black beans (200g/7oz/1¼ cups), well rinsed

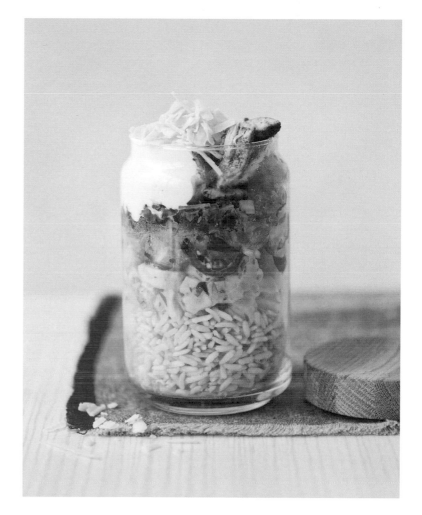

Heat a griddle pan until very hot, add the marinated chicken or vegetable and cook until lovely and charred.

To fill your jar, add the cooked and cooled rice first, followed by the guacamole and salsa, reserving some of the juice from it. Add the chicken or vegetable and the black beans. Pour over the remaining salsa juices, then top with the sour cream and grated cheese. This keeps well overnight in the refrigerator. You can keep it all in the jar or you can keep each part, except for the guacamole, separately for a few days. The guacamole needs to be made as close to eating as possible to keep it fresh and vibrant.

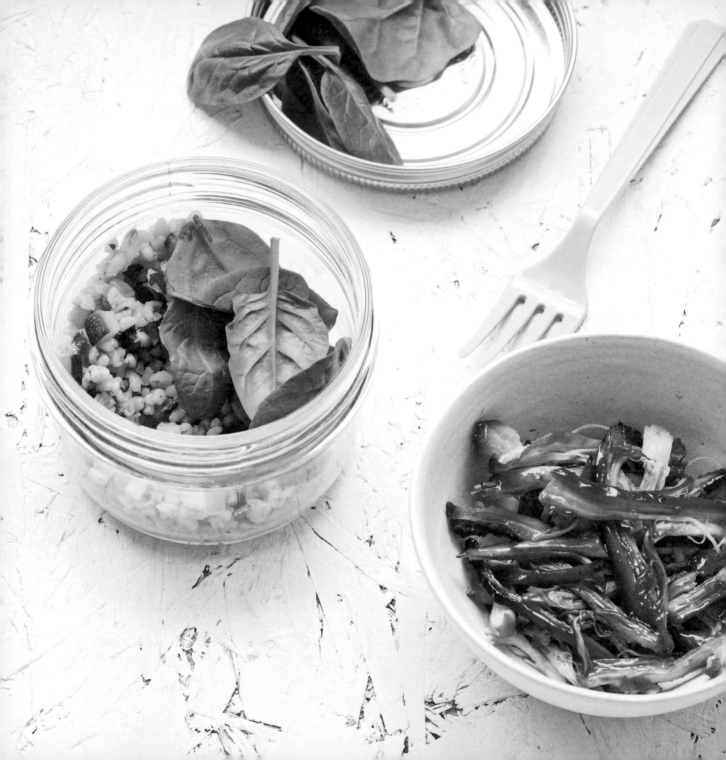

STICKY CHICKEN AND BULGUR WHEAT

INGREDIENTS

Makes 1 x 700ml/25fl oz jar
Keeps: 3–4 days

2 boneless, skinless chicken
   thighs
2 tbsp soy sauce
2 tbsp honey
1 chilli (chile), deseeded if desired
   and finely sliced
1 garlic clove, finely sliced
75g/2¾oz/scant ½ cup bulgur
   wheat
250ml/9fl oz/generous 1 cup
   vegetable stock
1 tbsp olive oil
1 courgette (zucchini), diced
½ red onion, diced
small handful of flat-leaf parsley
salt and freshly ground black
   pepper

This is my absolute go to when it comes to quick chicken dinners. The super-easy marinade makes the chicken so lovely and tender – it's a total winner and I use it for everything, such as stir-fries, soups, salads and, of course, this awesome filling bulgur wheat jar. Bulgur wheat takes on flavour very well, so add any vegetables you particularly like to bulk it out but don't forget those roasting juices, as they make all the difference.

Pop the chicken thighs, soy sauce, honey, chilli and garlic in a bowl, cover with clingfilm (plastic wrap) and leave to marinate in the refrigerator for as long as you can – overnight is ideal.

To make the bulgur wheat side, put the bulgur wheat and stock into a pan and bring to a simmer, then cover with a lid and cook for 12–15 minutes until the bulgur is soft and cooked through. Drain if there is any excess stock and set aside.

In the same pan, heat the olive oil, then add the courgette and onion and gently soften for 2 minutes. Add the bulgur wheat and fold through, adding salt and pepper as you wish. Remove from the heat and leave to cool.

When the bulgur wheat mixture is cool, mix through the parsley, then place in the bottom of your jar.

If you would like to bake the chicken, preheat the oven to 180°C/350°F/Gas mark 4 or preheat the grill (broiler). Grill (broil) the thighs for about 10 minutes, turning once, or bake for 25 minutes, or until the juices run clear. The honey will seem like it's burning but this caramelisation tastes delicious once they are done so don't panic. Shred the chicken thighs over the bulgur wheat in the jar and pour in any cooking juices for an added boost of flavour.

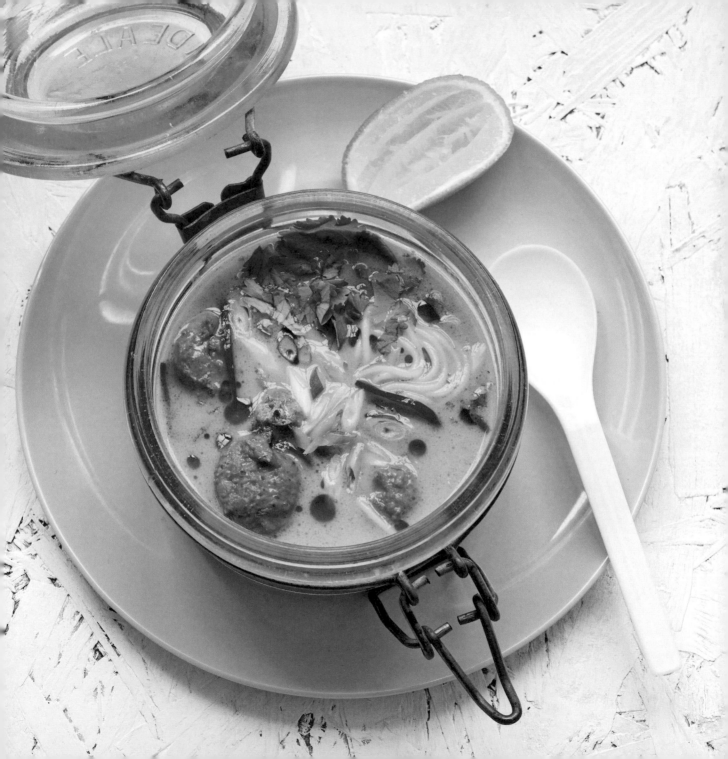

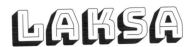

LAKSA

INGREDIENTS

Makes 1 x 700ml/25fl oz jar
Keeps: 3 days

For the prawn balls
100g/3½oz raw king prawns
   (jumbo shrimp)
1 tbsp Thai red curry paste
small handful of coriander
   (cilantro), stalks only

For the broth
small handful of vermicelli rice
   noodles
1 tsp coconut oil
100g/3½oz any sliced veg, such
   as cabbage, spinach or broccoli
2cm/¾in piece of fresh ginger,
   peeled
½ red chilli (chile), deseeded if
   desired
⅓ tsp ground turmeric
2 spring onions (scallions), finely
   chopped
2 kaffir lime leaves (dried is fine)
400ml/14fl oz can coconut milk
300ml/10fl oz/1¼ cups fish stock
1 tbsp sesame oil
1 tbsp fish sauce
1 tbsp soy sauce
1 tsp palm or light brown sugar
grated zest and juice of 1 lime
small handful of coriander
   (cilantro), leaves only, to garnish

There are so many awesome versions of laksa, but my favourite has to be the super-spiced and flavour-packed coconut milk ones. Eaten in Indonesia, Malaysia and Southern Thailand, thin vermicelli noodles are a perfect hidden ingredient as they soak up all the lovely flavour from the broth. You can pile any type of veg you fancy on top of the noodles and these awesome prawn balls bobbing in the broth. They take seconds to make and give some real sustenance to this otherwise light and fragrant dish.

Soak the noodles in a bowl of cold water for 15 minutes, then drain and set aside.

Start with the prawn balls, place the prawns, curry paste and coriander stalks in a food processer and pulse until combined but still quite chunky. Using wet hands, scoop the mixture out and shape into little balls – you should make around eight. Place on a plate, cover with clingfilm (plastic wrap)and chill in the refrigerator until the broth is ready.

Heat the coconut oil in a pan, add the vegetables, ginger, chilli, turmeric and spring onions and fry for 2 minutes. Add the kaffir lime leaves, coconut milk, stock, sesame oil, fish sauce, soy sauce and palm sugar to taste and simmer for 15 minutes. After 5 minutes, add the prawn balls and turn constantly to ensure they are cooked all the way through. Add the soaked noodles and stir through. Add the grated lime zest and juice, then carefully pour the laksa into your jar. Leave to cool, then tear up the coriander leaves and scatter over the top. Reheat over a low heat to ensure you don't overcook the prawn balls.

SHREDDED SPROUTS WITH PANCETTA AND WALNUT SLAW

INGREDIENTS

Makes 1 x 700ml/25fl oz jar
Keeps: 4 days (without dressing)
or 2 days (with dressing)

150g/5¼oz Brussels sprouts
1 small red onion
1 green eating apple
juice of ½ lemon
small handful of walnut pieces
100g/3½oz smoked pancetta
cubes (optional)

For the dressing
juice of ½ lemon
1 tsp maple syrup
1 tsp red wine vinegar
2 tbsp walnut oil
1 tsp Dijon mustard
1 small garlic clove, very finely
chopped
½ tsp each of sea salt and
freshly ground black pepper

Don't freak out if you're a sprouts hater – having them raw is a totally different experience! It's almost like a slaw in its texture with a lovely crunch and a sweet-sharp dressing. If you have a mandoline, that's awesome as it lets you get super-thin slices, but if your knife skills are up to it, you can also just chop them very finely instead. The pancetta is, of course, optional but its wonderful smoky flavour pairs with the maple syrup in the dressing really well, so definitely give it a go if you can.

Start by making the dressing, add all the ingredients to a small jar, cover with the lid and shake well until everything is combined. Leave at room temperature until the rest of your jar is ready to go.

Using a mandoline or knife, shred the Brussels sprouts into thin slices. Do the same with the red onion. Set both aside.

Grate the apple and toss in the lemon juice to ensure it doesn't go brown, then set aside.

Dry-fry the walnut pieces in a small frying pan (skillet) until they are nice and toasty, then remove from the pan and dry-fry the pancetta cubes, if using, until crispy.

Once everything is ready, it's time to layer up. Place the Brussels sprouts and onion slices into the bottom of your jar, followed by the apple, then the pancetta, if using, and finally, the walnuts. Pour in the dressing, pop the lid on and shake up to ensure everything's well coated. This one holds up quite well with the dressing on, even overnight but if you're making a couple of days ahead, keep it off and mix together just before you're ready to eat.

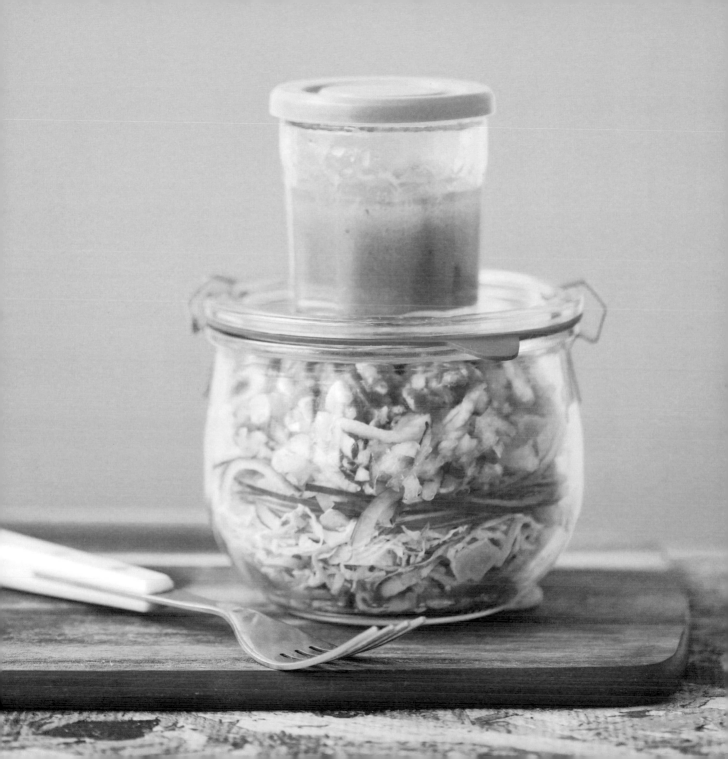

ASIAN NOODLE SOUP

INGREDIENTS

Makes 1 x 500ml/18fl oz jar
Keeps: 5 days

150g/5¼oz cooked chicken,
    prawns (shrimp) or tofu
    (optional)

For the flavour base pastes
1 tsp Tom Yum paste
1 tsp miso paste
1 tsp grated ginger
1 tsp bouillon powder

OR
1 tsp miso paste
1 tsp crunchy peanut butter
1 tsp Sriracha hot sauce
1 tsp grated ginger
1 tsp bouillon powder

For the vegetables
2 pak choi (bok choy) leaves
1 carrot
¼ red (bell) pepper
handful of beansprouts
small handful of edamame beans
1 spring onion (scallion)

small handful of coriander
    (cilantro)

For the noodles
small nest of instant ramen
    noodles
½ packet of cooked udon
    noodles
1 courgette (zucchini), spiralised
    or cut into strips with a peeler

With a chill in the air, there's nothing more warming than a spicy fragrant noodle soup. This is the easiest, healthiest and tastiest 'pot-noodle' you will ever make. It's important to mix your flavour base pastes well with the water and noodles when you come to finish off the soup. Try and cut your veg to all the same size if you can, as this makes them cook at the same rate and should give you a perfectly crunchy yet tender vibe to all the colourful veg. Anything goes with these guys so get creative and matchstick up any veg you have in the refrigerator.

First, make your flavour base paste. Mix all the ingredients together until smooth. Add anything you love and leave out anything you are not a fan of.

Next, prep all the vegetables. Cut them all into similar-sized matchsticks – we want everything to cook easily but still have a bit of a crunch. Small vegetables, such as beansprouts don't need chopping so don't worry about them. Now, it's time to layer up. Start with the flavour base, then add the noodles, cooked chicken, prawns or tofu (if using) and a couple of layers of vegetables. Once the layers are about halfway up the jar, add some more of the flavour paste and continue to layer up with what you fancy, finishing with the spring onions and coriander. Pop the lid on and leave in the refrigerator until ready to eat.

About 15 minutes before eating, remove the jar from the refrigerator so it has time to warm up or if you're in a rush just run it under a warm tap. Boil the kettle and slowly pour enough water to reach the top. Stir gently and pop the lid on for 5 minutes so all the ingredients heat up. Stir to mix all the flavours together and enjoy.

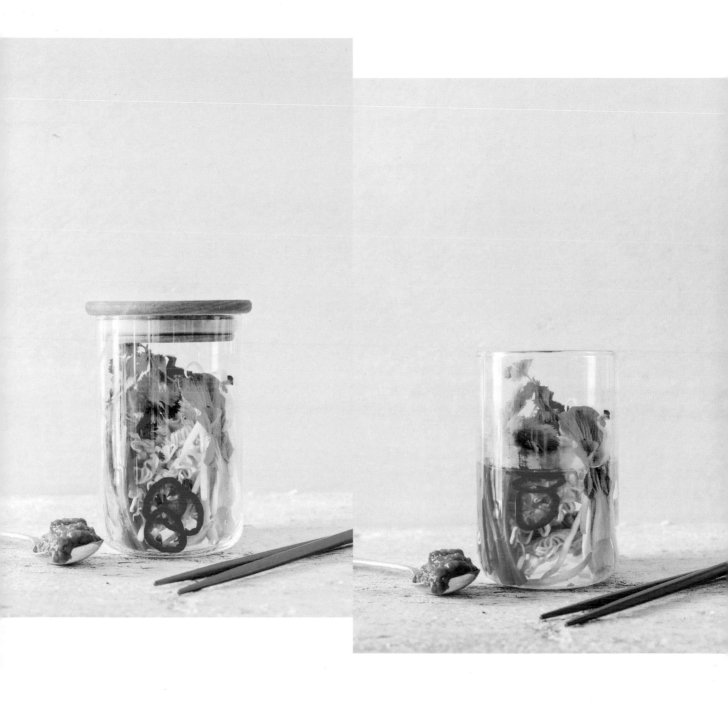

LAYERED MEDITERRANEAN FALAFEL SALAD WITH LEMON TAHINI DRESSING

INGREDIENTS

Makes 1 x 700ml/25fl oz jar
Keeps: 4 days (without dressing)

For the falafel
½ can chickpeas (200g/7oz/
  1½ cups), rinsed and dried
½ can mixed beans
  (200g/7oz/1¼ cups), rinsed
  and dried
grated zest and juice of ½ lemon
1 tsp harissa paste
1 tsp pomegranate ketchup,
  such as Aphrodite's (see recipe
  introduction)
2 garlic cloves
½ tsp allspice
1 tsp ground cumin
2 tbsp gram (chickpea) flour or
  plain (all-purpose) flour
1 tsp gluten-free baking powder
large pinch of salt
small bunch each of flat-leaf
  parsley and coriander (cilantro)
1 tbsp olive oil, for cooking

For the salad
2 tbsp olive oil
a pinch of sea salt
1 tsp dried mint
12 cherry or 2 large tomatoes,
  chopped

Pomegranate ketchup is something of a revelation to me – the sticky sweet beauty of pomegranates mixed with the tanginess of tomatoes gives these falafel a flavour that's out of this world. If you can't find any then a good thick tomato purée (paste) mixed with some pomegranate molasses would work well too, but if you can, it's seriously worth investing in a jar. Once you have done, you will find yourself using it for everything. My current obsession is it slathered on a cracker with a big hunk of Cheddar – tasty! The dressing in this salad is heavy on the garlic to balance the rest of the dish, but you can always use one clove if you are worried about breathing on everyone in the afternoon!

To make the falafel, put all the ingredients, except the olive oil, into a food processor and blitz to a smooth paste.

Meanwhile, to make the salad, mix the olive oil, sea salt and dried mint together in a bowl, add the chopped tomatoes and red onion and toss until coated. Set aside.

For the dressing, mix all the ingredients together in a bowl and set aside.

Using wet hands, shape the falafel mixture into small disks – you should get around eight. Heat the olive oil in a frying pan (skillet) over a low heat and fry the falafels for 5–8 minutes.

1 red onion, chopped
1 romaine lettuce,
    chopped
50g/1¾oz feta cheese,
    crumbled

**For the lemon tahini
dressing**
3 tbsp plain yogurt
2 garlic cloves, very
    finely chopped
2 tsp tahini paste
grated zest and juice
    of ½ lemon
sea salt

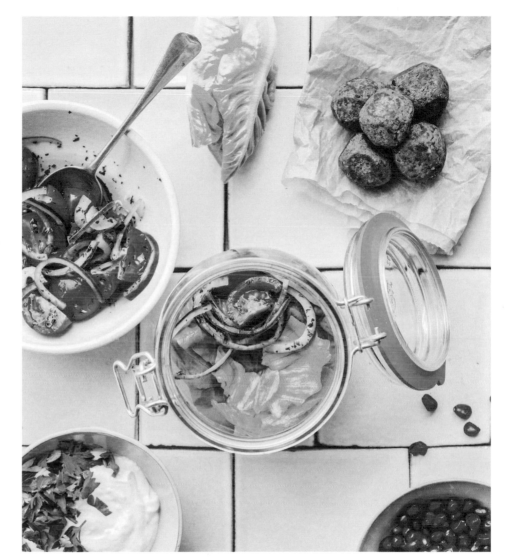

Place the lettuce in the bottom of your jar, then pile some of the tomato and onion mix on top. Add some of the dressing, then add a layer of falafel, followed by some feta. Repeat until you reach the top of the jar. Pop the lid on and store in the refrigerator until you are ready to eat. These are best eaten on the day they are made, but you can always put the dressing in another container and add it just before serving to keep the lettuce crisp.

ROAST BEEF AND BEET SALAD

INGREDIENTS

Makes 1 x 700ml/25fl oz jar
Keeps: 3 days

250g/9oz new potatoes
1 tbsp olive oil
½ tsp each of sea salt and
    freshly ground black pepper
1 beetroot (beet), skin on
1 small red onion
1 tbsp olive oil
1 thyme sprig
2 garlic cloves, unpeeled
4 roast beef slices (topside is
    great)
1 handful of watercress and
    spinach
2 tbsp pumpkin seeds

For the dressing
3 tbsp sour cream or crème
    fraîche
1 tbsp grated horseradish
1 tsp olive oil
squeeze of lemon juice
½ tsp each of sea salt and
    freshly ground black pepper

This jar (pictured on page 31) is perfect for a Monday lunch to use up all your leftovers from a lovely Sunday roast. Roast beef is my absolute favourite – lovely and pink in the middle makes it even more delicious the following day, as it stays beautifully soft. Leftover roast potatoes are an easy bottom layer but as there aren't always any left, these little new potatoes with sour cream make a great start to the jar. If you can't find fresh horseradish, the horseradish in a jar is great to use too. Don't be afraid to add more veg – how much of a roast dinner you would like this to be is completely up to you!

Preheat the oven to 180°C/350°F/Gas mark 4.

Toss the new potatoes in the olive oil and salt and pepper, then place on a baking tray and set aside.

Roughly chop the beetroot and red onion and place on another baking tray. Add the olive oil, thyme and garlic to the beetroot and red onion and toss until coated. Place in the hot oven. After 45 minutes, add the potatoes to the oven and continue cooking for a further 45 minutes.

While the veg is cooking, make your dressing by shaking all the ingredients up in a small jar and leaving in the fridge until using.

When cooked, press the potatoes down with the back of a spoon to crush lightly and pop into the bottom of your jar. Add the dressing, then follow this with the wonderful purple beetroot and onions and all their cooking juices. Squeeze the insides of the garlic cloves into the jar, then add the roast beef slices on top. Top with the watercress and spinach and a sprinkling of pumpkin seeds to keep them crunchy!

LENTIL STEW

INGREDIENTS

Makes 2 x 500ml/18fl oz jars
Keeps: 4 days

1 tbsp olive oil
1 onion, diced
1 carrot, diced
1 celery stick, chopped
1 garlic clove, crushed
200g/7oz squash or pumpkin
150g/5¼oz/¾ cup green lentils
½ tsp ground turmeric
½ tsp ground cinnamon
½ tsp ground cumin
½ tsp cayenne pepper
400g/14oz can chopped
   tomatoes
300ml/10fl oz/1¼ cups
   vegetable stock

Warming up a jar of stew is so lovely and comforting on a cold lunch break. Lentils are so cheap and when squash season is in town, this jar comes in at a crazily low price per portion. Bulk it out with your favourite veg or add more lentils if you really dig them – just make sure to adjust the liquid quantities accordingly. When you are reheating the stew you also may need to add a splash of water to loosen it.

Heat the olive oil in a large pan, add the onion, carrot, celery and garlic and fry for 4 minutes to soften. Add the squash and lentils and fry for a further 2 minutes. Add the spices and stir well so all the spices coat the vegetables. Add the tomatoes and stock and stir again, then cover with a lid and let bubble over a medium heat for 30 minutes until the lentils are tender.

Divide the stew between your jars and leave to cool to room temperature before covering with the lids and storing in the refrigerator until ready to eat.

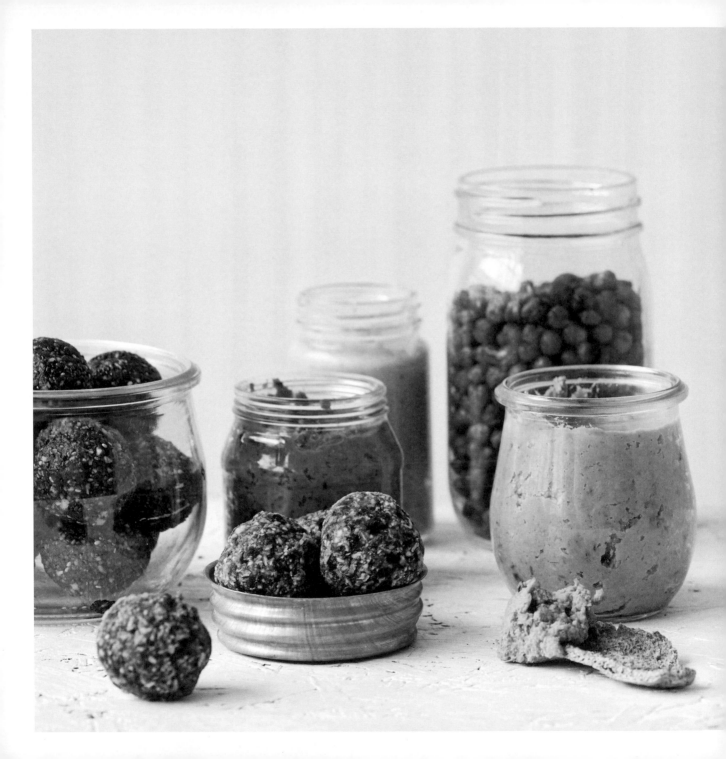

SNACKS

If you feel sluggish or tired mid-morning or afternoon, then these snacks are a great way to keep you going. They are super-tasty and can fend off those sweet or salty cravings without you reaching for the shop-bought snacks. I make a couple of these over the weekend and keep them on my desk to dive into when I need a boost.

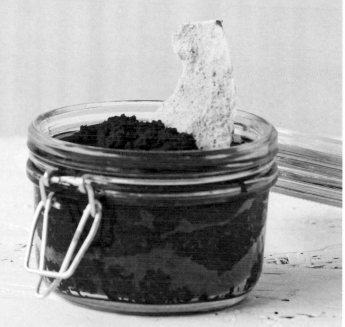

SPICY CRUNCHY CHICKPEAS

INGREDIENTS

Makes 1 x 350ml/9fl oz jar
Keeps: 2 weeks

400g/14oz can chickpeas,
    drained and rinsed
3 tbsp olive oil
sea salt and freshly ground black
    pepper
½ tsp seasoning, such as smoked
    paprika, cayenne pepper,
    onion or garlic powder, wasabi
    powder

This is a super-simple snack and the only fiddly bit is right at the beginning, which can be done while having a chat with your housemates. Get creative with your seasonings and even try a few different ones in the same jar for a surprise in every bite!

Preheat the oven to 160°C/325°F/Gas mark 3.

Get your peel on! Start by pinching each chickpea between your index finger and thumb and remove the opaque outer jacket of each one. This is worth doing to get them super-crunchy.

Spread the chickpeas out on a baking tray and place them straight in the hot oven for 20 minutes until light golden brown. Remove from the oven and add the olive oil and salt and pepper, then return to the oven and continue to roast for 15–20 minutes until they are super-crunchy.

Once cooked and cooled, add whatever seasoning you like and pop in your jar – cayenne pepper always gives me a mid-afternoon boost. Seal up and store at room temperature.

PITTA CHIPS

INGREDIENTS

Makes 1 x 500ml/18fl oz jar
Keeps: 5 days

2 tbsp olive oil
1 tsp paprika
1 tsp onion salt
2 pitta breads

These little triangles of joy are so easy to make at home and way better for you than shop-bought crisps. Another plus is that you can make them your own! They last for about a week so make a big batch and season them with different spices and herbs to keep you going for an awesome savoury hit when you need to fight lunch cravings.

Preheat the oven to 180°C/350°F/Gas mark 4 and pop a baking tray into the oven to heat up.

Whisk the olive oil, paprika and onion salt together in a small bowl. Split the pittas as they naturally do and cut each side into a few triangles. Coat lightly in the oil and spices and spread out on the hot baking tray - thick sides on one half and thin on the other. Bake the chips in the hot oven for 6–8 minutes for the thin sides and 10 minutes for the thick sides. Leave to cool, then store in your jar.

VEGETABLE HUMMUS

INGREDIENTS

Makes 1 x 500ml/18fl oz jar
Keeps: 7 days

200g/7oz can chickpeas
   (garbanzo beans), drained but
   liquid reserved
1 tsp tahini
1 garlic clove, very finely
   chopped
1 tsp sea salt
grated zest and juice of ½ lemon
3–4 tbsp extra virgin olive oil
paprika, for sprinkling
vegetable crudités, to serve

Hummus is one of the yummiest snacks around and without a doubt, one of the simplest. The basic recipe is just a handful of ingredients and the additions are just as easy to rustle up to make a few different versions. I have included a few of my favourites, but if you have a veg you can't get enough of, just roast it to intensify the flavour and add it along with your chickpeas for a delicious twist.

Place all the ingredients, except the olive oil and paprika, into a food processor and pulse a few times to get started. Continue to blend, adding 2 tbsp of the reserved chickpea liquid and enough olive oil to come to a consistency you like. Sprinkle with paprika and a drizzle of extra olive oil if you like, then pop in your jar. Serve with a selection of crudités for the perfect afternoon snack.

VARIATIONS

Beetroot and Mint Hummus
Preheat the oven to 160°C/325°F/Gas mark 3. Roast 200g/7oz beetroot (beet) in olive oil and salt and freshly ground black pepper wrapped in foil in the hot oven for 40–50 minutes until tender. Whizz the roasted beetroot with the chickpeas, 2 tsp dried mint and a large handful of fresh mint until smooth.

Red Onion Hummus
Preheat the oven to 160°C/325°F/Gas mark 3. Roast 1 large red onion with 2 tbsp olive oil, salt and freshly ground black pepper in the hot oven for 30 minutes. Add to the chickpea mix in the food processor after they have had a quick blitz and continue whizzing until smooth.

Sun-drenched Tomato and Basil Hummus
Add 150g/5¼oz sun-drenched tomatoes to the chickpeas in the food processor and whizz with a small handful of basil until smooth.

NUT BUTTER AND FRUIT CRISPS

INGREDIENTS

Makes 1 x 250ml/9fl oz jar
Keeps: Butter up to 3 weeks in
refrigerator and crisps up to
4 days in a sealed jar

For the butter
200g/7oz/1½ cups raw almonds,
skin on
1 tsp sea salt
2 tbsp maple syrup

For the fruit crisps
1 apple
1 pear
½ tsp ground cinnamon (optional)

TOP TIP!

Don't panic. It can seem like
forever for nut butter to work
in the food processor but just
keep going. It will look like
breadcrumbs, then like cookie
dough and then like it will never
come together but the trick is
just to keep going. Make sure
your food processor can handle
it and if it feels like it's getting
hot, take a 10-minute break and
come straight back to it.

If you're feeling adventurous then making your own nut butters can be
a great experiment to crack on with over the weekend. The weight of
the nuts you roast, becomes pretty much exactly the amount of butter
you're left with at the end, so see what size jars you have and work it out
accordingly. I love having a good 3–4cm/1¼–1½in deep layer at the bottom
of mine and layering the fruit crisps up so it's all there ready to go.

Preheat the oven to 180°C/350°F/Gas mark 4.

For the butter, pop the almonds on a baking tray and roast in the hot oven
for 10 minutes until they smell heavenly. Remove and leave to cool.

Reduce the oven temperature to 100°C/212°F/lowest possible Gas mark.

For the fruit crisps, a mandoline will make it much easier to achieve super-
thin slices, which makes the crisping up process a lot faster, otherwise
you can use a sharp knife. Slice the apple and pear as thin as you can and
spread out over a baking tray, dust them with the cinnamon, if using, and
bake in the hot oven for about 45 minutes, or until most of the moisture
has left them. Leave to cool and crisp up on the tray.

To finish the butter, pop the nuts, sea salt and maple syrup into a food
processor and whizz on high speed for 5 minutes. Scrap the bowl down
properly and whizz again for a further 5 minutes. Scrape the bowl down
for a final time and whizz for another 5 minutes or so or until it's smooth.
Pop the butter into your jar. Decant the butter and eat with your fruit
crisps as a delicious snack during the week.

ENERGY BALLS

INGREDIENTS

Each recipe makes 8 balls
Keeps: 7 days

I have the biggest sweet tooth in the world and needed to try and find something that would satisfy my need for a pudding after lunch and dinner, but not be totally full of the bad stuff. These guys are refined sugar- and gluten-free and all the more tasty for it.

CHOCOLATE ORANGE

100g/3½oz/¾ cup pitted dates
75g/2¾oz/½ cup almonds,
   skins on
75g/2¾oz/scant ⅓ cup cashew
   nuts
2 tbsp chia seeds
1 tsp coconut oil, melted
3 tsp cocoa powder, plus extra
   for rolling
2 tsp orange extract

Soak the dates in a heatproof bowl of boiling water for 10 minutes.

Blitz the nuts a little in a food processor, then add the soaked dates, chia seeds, coconut oil, cocoa powder and orange extract and pulse to get it started if you need to, then continue to blend, scraping the bowl down regularly to ensure it's a nice even mix. Using wet hands, roll the mixture into eight balls, then roll them in the extra cocoa until coated. Chill in the refrigerator for 8 hours, or freeze for 1 hour if you are in a rush. They are also delicious totally frozen as mini choc-ice type things.

PISTACHIO, COCONUT AND CRANBERRY (FESTIVE EDITION!)

100g/3½oz/¾ cup pitted dates
75g/2¾oz/1 cup desiccated
   (dry unsweetened shredded)
   coconut
3 tsp coconut oil, melted
75g/2¾oz/½ cup unsalted
   pistachios
50g/1¾oz/scant ½ cup dried
   cranberries

Soak the dates in a heatproof bowl of boiling water for 10 minutes.

Blitz the coconut in a food processor until it is super-fine; almost like a flour. Add the soaked dates, coconut oil and pistachios and pulse until it comes together. Add the cranberries and blitz for a little longer. Using wet hands, roll the mixture into eight balls. Chill in the refrigerator for a few hours or freeze for 1 hour.

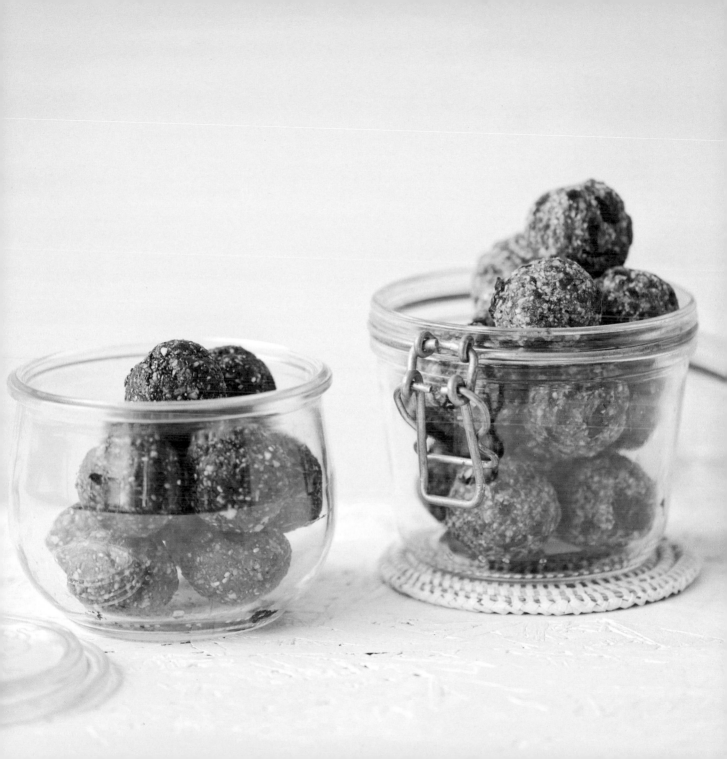

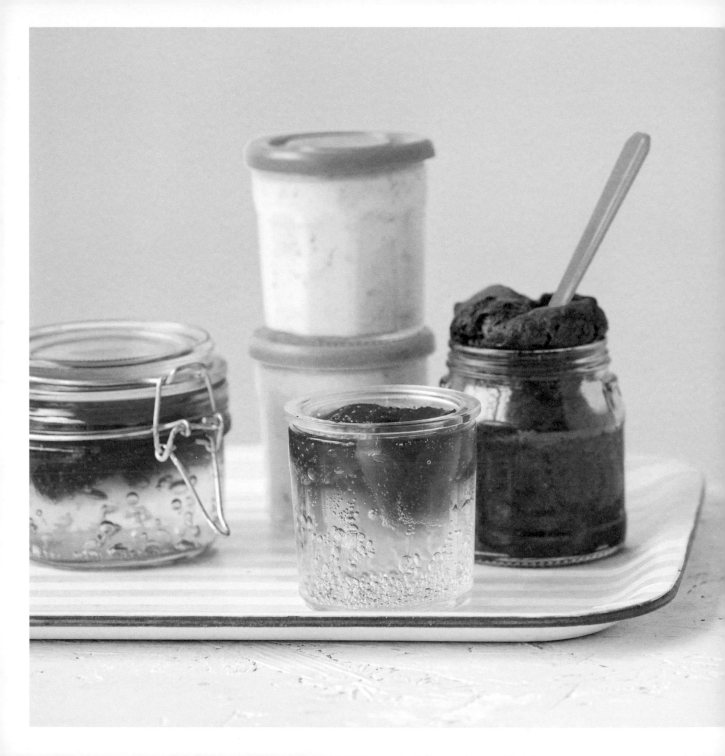

DESSERTS

Tiny jars make everything cuter. These little guys are perfect as a post-lunch treat or for a gathering of friends when you fancy something a bit extra. Jars are a perfect pudding vessel as you can chill them, bake them and even freeze them – all with easy portioning already done for you!

ORANGE AND GINGER POSSET JARS

INGREDIENTS

Makes 4 x 100ml/3½fl oz jars
Keeps: 3 days

350ml/12fl oz/1½ cups double
(heavy) cream
3 pieces of stem (preserved)
ginger, chopped
75ml/2½ fl oz/5 tbsp stem
(preserved) ginger syrup from
the jar
2 tsp ground ginger
grated zest and juice of 1 large
orange

These little cuties are the perfect post-dinner pick me up. Rich enough to feel satisfying but small enough to make you not feel too guilty! Orange and ginger is a match made in heaven and instead of your summery lemon posset vibes, these have a much more autumnal flavour. When they are in season, I love to use blood oranges for their distinctive flavour and colour but these are equally great all year round with regular oranges.

Place the cream, stem (preserved) ginger, ginger syrup and ground ginger in a pan over a low heat and bring to a gentle simmer. Let bubble for 2 minutes – it may turn a more golden colour and thicken but don't panic, keep your eye on it so it doesn't boil over. Remove from the heat after 2–3 minutes and add the grated orange zest and juice. Stir until it is well incorporated, then pour into your jars. Leave to set at room temperature before placing in the refrigerator for 4–6 hours, or preferably overnight.

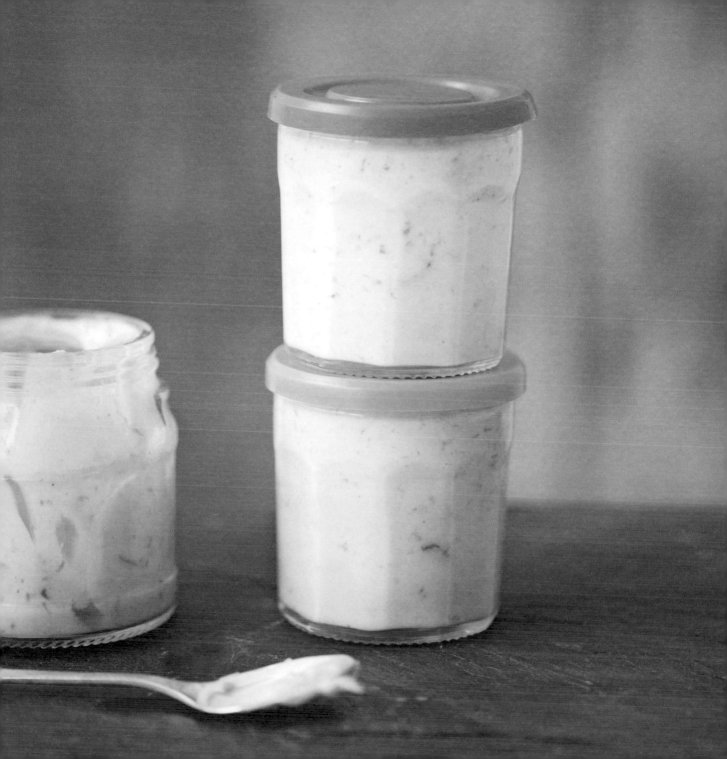

LADY GREY PANNA COTTA

INGREDIENTS

Makes 4 x 100ml/3½fl oz jars
Keeps: 4 days

3 sheets leaf gelatine
250ml/9fl oz/1 cup whole milk
250ml/9fl oz/generous 1 cup
    double (heavy) cream
2 Lady Grey teabags
grated zest of 1 lemon
berries, to serve (optional)

Panna cotta is a classic dessert but very rarely strays away from vanilla as its main flavour. I'm obsessed with all things tea and in particular, Lady Grey. Its beautiful notes of bergamot and light citrus peel works wonderfully with the richness of the cream making for a refreshing yet decadent dessert. You don't need to eat much of these, so they are a perfect after dinner treat.

Soak the gelatine leaves in a small bowl of cold water for a few minutes to soften.

Bring the milk, cream and teabags to a low simmer in a pan over a low heat. Make sure it doesn't boil over. Let bubble for 2 minutes, then remove from the heat.

Squeeze out the excess water from the gelatine leaves and add them, one at a time, to the pan, stirring well to dissolve them after each addition. When they have all melted, squeeze out the teabags and discard.

Pour the mixture into your small jars and leave in the refrigerator for 4-6 hours. Serve with berries, if you like.

BANANA, PEANUT BUTTER AND MAPLE "NICE" CREAM

INGREDIENTS

Makes 1 x 250ml/9fl oz jar
Keeps: up to 1 month, frozen

3 very ripe bananas, frozen
125g/4½oz/½ cup crunchy
   peanut butter
100g/3½oz/1/3 cup maple syrup
2 tsp vanilla bean paste
1 tsp sea salt
1 tsp ground cinnamon (optional)
small handful of chopped pecans

I don't make a habit of tricking those I'm feeding but with this it was too easy. Frozen bananas are the vegan ice cream equivalent of the best cream in the world! It's almost impossible to believe that there's no dairy in this yummy jar. The creativity you could have with this as a base is extraordinary. Go wild with berries or keep it simple with some salted caramel. This is a true pudding fiend's delight! It may seem odd having a weight for the maple syrup but I stick my whole food processor bowl on the scales and weigh it all in there – it saves so much time and washing up.

Whizz all the ingredients, except the pecans, in a food processor until smooth. If you have not used frozen bananas, pop this wonderful mix in your jars then place them into the freezer for 45–60 minutes to harden. Stir through the pecans and go to town!

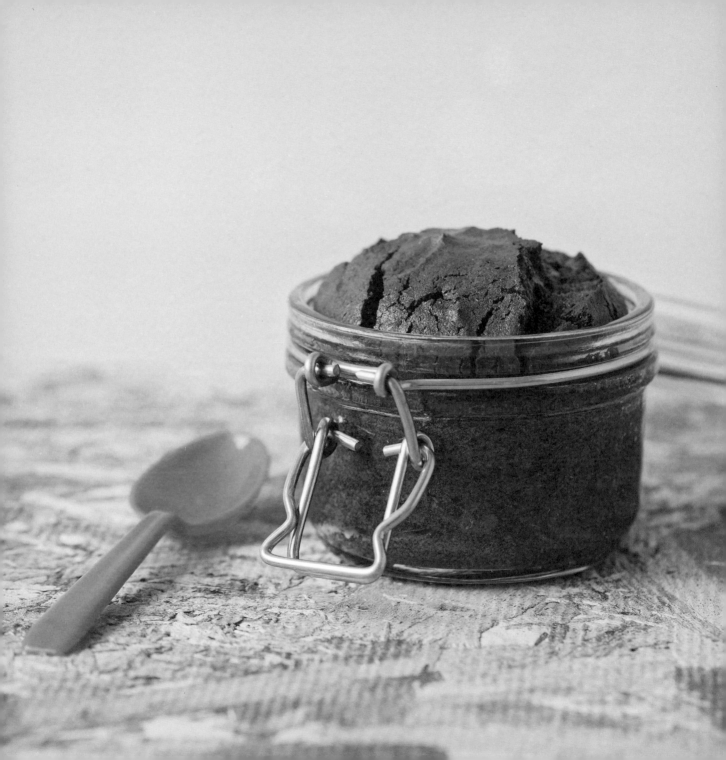

HOT CHOCOLATE MOUSSE JARS

INGREDIENTS

Makes 4 x 250ml/9fl oz
    heatproof jars
Keeps: 4 days

130g/4½oz dark (bittersweet)
    chocolate (at least 80% cocoa
    solids), broken into pieces
130g/4½oz/9 tbsp unsalted
    butter
4 eggs, separated
130g/4½oz/about ⅔ cup soft
    light brown sugar
2 tbsp coffee (can be instant
    powder)
50g/1¾oz/½ cup cocoa powder
1 tsp vanilla bean paste
½ tsp fine sea salt

As any chocoholic will tell you, anything with a molten middle is infinitely better and these are no exception. They rise beautifully like a soufflé yet have the most indulgent middle that makes them at their best straight out of the oven. The recipe itself, however, does lend itself to being very similar to a flourless chocolate cake, meaning that these jars can last and last! It's almost a different pudding entirely a day later, but is just as yummy eaten hot or cold with a dollop of crème fraîche on top.

Preheat the oven to 160°C/325°F/Gas mark 3.

First, melt the chocolate and butter together until they are smooth (either in the microwave at 30 second intervals or in a bowl over a pan of simmering water), then set aside.

Next, whisk the egg whites until they have tripled in volume and stiff peaks have formed. Transfer them to another bowl, then whisk the egg yolks and brown sugar together until doubled in volume and the whisk leaves a trail across the surface. Add the coffee, cocoa, vanilla and sea salt to the yolks mix and whisk well until it is all incorporated. Gently pour in the melted chocolate and butter mixture, then add one-third of the egg whites into the yolks and mix gently to loosen. Fold the rest of the whites in delicately so as not to lose the air you have worked hard to get in there!

Pour the mixture into your jars, pop on a baking tray and bake in the hot oven for 18 minutes.

LEMON CRUNCH POTS

INGREDIENTS

Makes 4 x 100ml/3½fl oz
    heatproof jars
Keeps: Eat straightaway

For the base
100g/3½oz/1 cup gluten-free
    oats
100g/3½oz/¾ cup raw almonds,
    skin on
½ tsp sea salt
2 tbsp maple syrup
65–75g/2¼–2¾oz/scant 1/3–
    generous 1/3 cup coconut oil,
    melted

For the topping
100g/3½oz/generous ¾ cup
    cashew nuts
200g/7oz block coconut cream,
    warmed in a bowl of hot water
    until soft
2 tbsp cornflour (cornstarch)
½ tsp sea salt
grated zest and juice of 3 lemons
4 tbsp maple syrup, plus extra
    to taste

If you are anything like me then lemon desserts hold a special place in your heart. The base of these pots is the nuttiest most delicious biscuit (cookie) you have ever had. Drizzled with very good-quality dark (bittersweet) chocolate would be more than enough for me but this coconut cream and lemon concoction on top takes it to another level. They don't keep very well so it's best to eat them straight from the oven or reheat them if you have made them a couple of hours ahead to keep the pudding lovely and fluffy.

Soak the cashew nuts for the topping in a bowl of cold water overnight, then drain.

The next day, preheat the oven to 175°C/350°F/Gas mark 4.

Blitz the oats, almonds and sea salt together in a food processor or blender until it forms very fine crumbs. Gradually add the maple syrup and melted coconut oil until it starts to come together like a dough. Press this into the bottom of your jars, place on a baking tray and bake in the hot oven for about 15-20 minutes until golden on top.

Add the soaked cashews to the clean food processor or blender, squeeze in the coconut cream (which should be all soft and melted), the cornflour, sea salt, grated lemon zest and juice and the maple syrup and blend until smooth, thick and creamy. Taste. If it's a little on the sharp side, add some more maple syrup until you reach the desired sweetness.

Pour the topping onto the cooked bases in the jars and return to the oven for about 20-25 minutes until just set – they should still have a little wobble in the centre. Devour instantly!

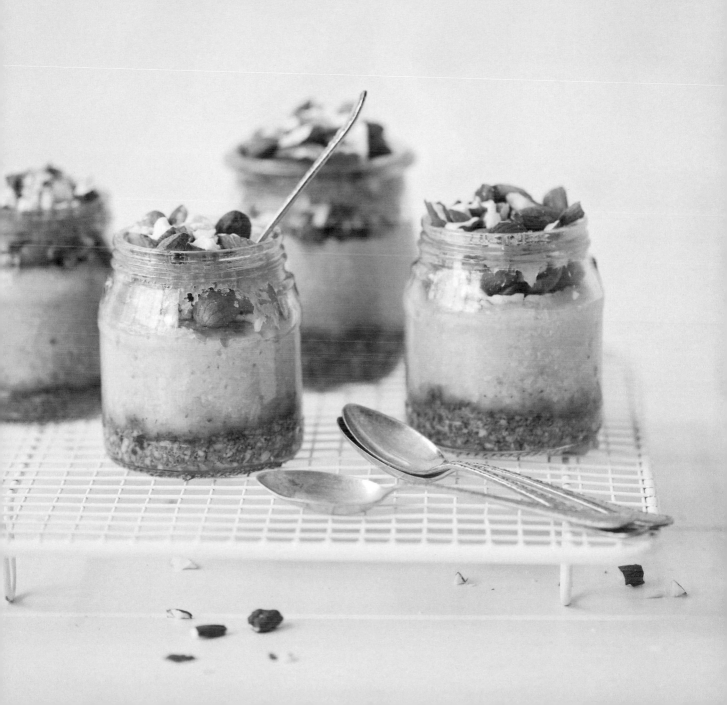

MEGA FRUIT CRUMBLE JARS

INGREDIENTS

Makes 4 x 250ml/9fl oz
   heatproof jars
Keeps: 3 days

6–8 plums
grated zest and juice of 1 orange
1 tbsp light soft brown sugar
1 star anise
1 punnet of blackberries
   (150g/5¼oz/1 cup)
1 tsp ground cinnamon
1 tsp ground nutmeg
1 tsp vanilla bean paste

For the crumble:
100g/3½oz/¾ cup plain
   (all-purpose) flour
100g/3½oz/7 tbsp cold unsalted
   butter, cubed
50g/1¾oz/¼ cup muscovado
   (soft brown) sugar
25g/1oz/¼ cup jumbo rolled oats
50g/1¾oz/⅓ cup pecans,
   chopped

Crumbles are just one of those puddings that instantly put a smile on your face. Everyone has a wonderful memory of a crumble – whether it's after an amazing Sunday roast or a great pub lunch, crumble is a sure-fire winner. Served individually in jars, these make sure everyone has some of the lovely crunchy topping you normally fight over! Spices for me in a crumble are non-negotiable and star anise works so well. Plums and blackberries are great bedfellows, but use whatever is in season. Make sure the fruit is flavoursome, so it can take the spices well. Mix it up and see what other combinations you can come up with!

Preheat the oven to 180°C/350°F/Gas mark 4.

Start by slicing each plum in half and removing the stone (pit). Pop the plum halves in a pan with the grated orange zest and juice, soft brown sugar and star anise. Pop a lid on and cook over a low heat for 10 minutes, or until the plums are soft. Add the blackberries, the remaining spices and the vanilla bean paste, then pop spoonfuls of the fruit into each jar.

To make the crumble, in a bowl, rub the flour and butter together with your fingertips until a rough crumb comes together. Stir through the muscovado (brown) sugar, oats and pecans until combined, then sprinkle all over the top of the fruit in your jars. Get it as thick as you like! Place the jars on a baking tray and bake in the hot oven for about 20–30 minutes, or until golden brown and crunchy. If the topping browns too quickly, pop foil over the top for the last 10 minutes or so. Serve straightaway as a hot pudding or enjoy it cold as the best of breakfasts in the morning!

FRUIT FIZZ JELLIES

INGREDIENTS

Makes 4 x 100ml/3½fl oz jars
(with a little spare)
Keeps: 3 days

250ml/9fl oz/generous 1 cup
    prosecco or pink lemonade
100g/3½oz/1 cup raspberries
3 leaves of gelatine
40g/1½oz/scant ¼ cup caster
    (superfine) sugar
200ml/7fl oz/scant 1 cup water

Light, fruity and fizzy, these jellies (pictured on page 66) are the perfect desserts for after any meal. Fresh summer berries are gorgeous when you can get them, but these are just as nice as a plain jelly. If you are not a drinker, use something such as pink lemonade or another fizzy cordial of your liking instead of the alcohol. It's important to keep everything chilled so the bubbles can stay suspended in the jelly and then burst on your tongue. Pop your jars and fruit in the refrigerator and make sure the prosecco is really cold by popping it in the freezer for an hour or so before making.

These jellies are so lovely for a little midweek indulgence after one of the lighter salads such as the Hot Smoked Salmon and Watercress Jar (see page 42), but they are also an easy to make-ahead dessert if you have people round for dinner.

Put your jars, prosecco or lemonade and raspberries into the refrigerator to chill.

Add a little cold water to a shallow dish, pop the gelatine leaves in side by side and leave to soften for a few minutes. Melt the sugar and measured water together in a pan over a medium heat, then bring to a gentle simmer. Cook for 2 minutes, then add the gelatine leaves, one at a time, and stir well to melt them. Remove the pan from the heat and leave to cool.

Remove your jars, prosecco and fruit from the refrigerator and stir the prosecco into the gelatine and sugar mixture until combined. Pour the mixture into a jug (pitcher), then pour into the jars. Add the raspberries and push them down so they are submerged. Leave to set in the refrigerator for 2–3 hours.

STOCKISTS

Amazon
www.amazon.co.uk
Useful online marketplace for
hard-to-find ingredients and
equipment.

Aphrodite's Food Ltd
Arches 370 and 371
Station Road
London E7 0AB
+44(0) 20 8534 8471
www.aphroditesfood.com/shop/
Small batch producer of
specialist Eastern Mediterranean
ingredients including
pomegranate ketchup. Stockists
across London, UK.

Booths
Central Office
Longridge Road
Ribbleton
Preston PR2 5BX
0800 221 8086
www.booths.co.uk
Good-quality produce sourced
from local suppliers in the north of
England.

Holland & Barrett
www.hollandbarrett.com
High street health-food store
with online shop and nationwide
delivery.

Lucy Bee
PO Box 214
Hertford
Hertfordshire SG14 2ZX
+44 (0)1992 537 874
www.lucybee.co
This is my favourite brand of
coconut oil and can be found in
supermarkets and online.

Ocado
www.ocado.com
Online supermarket for home
delivery.

Pip & Nut
www.pipandnut.com
This is my favourite brand of nut
butters, available direct and in
supermarkets nationwide.

Planet Organic
www.planetorganic.com
Wide range of organic foods.

Rude Health
www.rudehealth.com
Organic almond, coconut and rice
milks for dairy-free dishes.

Sainsbury's
www.sainsburys.co.uk
Supermarket selling fresh, quality
food and drink.

Tesco
www.tesco.com
Supermarket selling fresh, quality
food and drink.

Waitrose
www.waitrose.com
Supermarket selling fresh, quality
food and drink.

Whole Foods Market
www.wholefoodsmarket.com
Organic and whole foods stockist
of leading health food brands and
well-sourced produce.

INDEX

ACKNOWLEDGMENTS

For Uncle Phil – as sweet peas do always look so lovely in jars.

Firstly, I have to thank my parents, Juliet and Stuart. You both inspire me every day with how you approach life and how you always push me to do better and to enjoy the world around me. You have given me every foundation to do this and I hope you know how much I appreciate it.

To Rachel, who has been there for my highest of highs and lowest of lows. There is no one I would rather have been on this rollercoaster with and I am so lucky to have you and your never faltering belief in me. You make me a better person every day and this wouldn't have happened without you.

To Maxine and Bee, thank you for showing me that girl bosses can rock and that women supporting women is something that we all need and should aspire to have in our lives. We are stronger together and we can be awesome while doing it.

Finally, to the team at Pavilion. Emily for noticing something in me and believing that I could do this, Tory and Steph for all your help and guidance, Laura and Lee-May for your wicked design skills. This also couldn't have been possible without Charlie and her eye for style and Clare for her beautiful pictures. Together this has been an incredible experience and I'm so very grateful to be able to share it with all of you. Thank you.

First published in the United Kingdom in 2017 by
Pavilion
43 Great Ormond Street
London
WC1N 3HZ

Copyright © Pavilion Books Company Ltd 2017
Text copyright © Dominique Eloïse Alexander 2017

ISBN 978-1-91121-676-6

A CIP catalogue record for this book is available from the British Library.

10 9 8 7 6 5 4 3 2 1

Reproduction by Mission Productions Ltd., Hong Kong
Printed and bound by 1010 Printing International Ltd, China

This book can be ordered direct from the publisher
at www.pavilionbooks.com

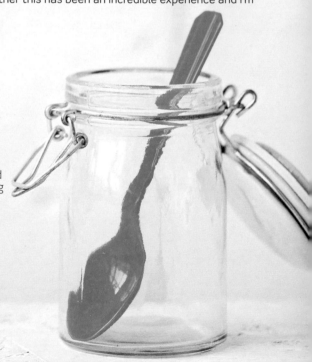